INTERMITTENT FASTING FOR WOMEN OVER 50

INTERMITTENT FASTING FOR WOMEN OVER 50

Every Burning Question About Weight Loss, Mental Health, Disease Prevention, Anti-Aging, and More: ANSWERED!

BRITNEY LYNCH

Copyright © Britney Lynch 2021 - All rights reserved.

The content contained within this book may not be reproduced, duplicated or transmitted without direct written permission from the author or the publisher.

Under no circumstances will any blame or legal responsibility be held against the publisher, or author, for any damages, reparation, or monetary loss due to the information contained within this book, either directly or indirectly.

Legal Notice:

This book is copyright protected. It is only for personal use. You cannot amend, distribute, sell, use, quote or paraphrase any part, or the content within this book, without the consent of the author or publisher.

Disclaimer Notice:

Please note the information contained within this document is for educational and entertainment purposes only. All effort has been executed to present accurate, up to date, reliable, complete information. No warranties of any kind are declared or implied. Readers acknowledge that the author is not engaged in the rendering of legal, financial, medical or professional advice. The content within this book has been derived from various sources. Please consult a licensed professional before attempting any techniques outlined in this book.

By reading this document, the reader agrees that under no circumstances is the author responsible for any losses, direct or indirect, that are incurred as a result of the use of the information contained within this document, including, but not limited to, errors, omissions, or inaccuracies.

CONTENTS

Introduction — 1

Chapter 1
UNDERSTANDING INTERMITTENT FASTING — 5

The History Behind Intermittent Fasting — 5

What is Intermittent Fasting and How Does it Work? — 6

Why Choose Intermittent Fasting Over Traditional Diets? — 7

Intermittent Fasting and Women Over 50 — 8

7 Myths About Intermittent Fasting: Debunked! — 9

Chapter 2
THE MANY BENEFITS OF INTERMITTENT FASTING — 13

How Intermittent Fasting Helps You Lose Weight — 13

Intermittent Fasting and Heart Health — 14

Intermittent Fasting and the Brain — 15

Intermittent Fasting and Alzheimer's — 16

How Does Fasting Boost Cognitive Functioning in Mice? — 17

Who Shouldn't Fast? 17

Chapter 3
AGING AND INTERMITTENT FASTING FOR OLDER WOMEN 23

How Does Aging Hamper Weight Loss in Women? 23

How Does Fasting Slow the Aging Process? 24

Fasting and Autophagy Explained 25

Tips for Transitioning to Intermittent Fasting Properly 27

Chapter 4
EIGHT OF THE MOST EFFECTIVE METHODS OF FASTING: EXPLAINED! 31

A Precautionary Word 31

The Crescendo Method 32

The Leangains or 16/8 Method 32

The 5/2 Method 33

Eat Stop Eat 34

The Warrior Diet 35

Alternate-Day Fasting 35

Spontaneous Meal Skipping 37

Overnight Fasting or 12-Hour Fasting 37

The Bottom Line 38

Chapter 5
EIGHT EFFECTIVE METHODS OF FASTING: GETTING STARTED WITH A COMPREHENSIVE GUIDE — 39

- Special Note for Women — 39
- The Crescendo Method — 40
- The Leangains or 16/8 Method — 42
- The 5:2 Method — 45
- Eat Stop Eat — 47
- The Warrior Diet — 49
- Alternate-Day Fasting — 52

Chapter 6
TIPS AND TRICKS FOR ACHIEVING INTERMITTENT FASTING SUCCESS — 57

- What Can I Expect When Starting to Fast? — 57
- How Do I Know I'm Fasting Correctly? — 58
- 17 Key Tips for Fasting Success — 58
- How to Avoid Emotional Eating — 63
- How to Avoid Fasting Side Effects — 65
- How Do I Track My Progress? — 68
- How to Maintain Intermittent Fasting — 69
- Foods to Eat While Fasting — 69
- Foods to Avoid While Fasting — 70

Chapter 7
40 INTERMITTENT FASTING QUALITY RECIPES FOR WEIGHT LOSS AND ANTI-AGING   71

- Orange and Apricot Quinoa   72
- Super Healthy Breakfast Burrito   74
- Savory Steel Cut Meal   76
- Pomegranate Yogurt   78
- Acai Breakfast Bowl   80
- Banana Flax Breakfast Muffins   82
- Mixed Berry and Banana Smoothie   84
- Superfood Oatmeal   86
- Anti-Inflammatory Superfood Turmeric Berry Smoothie   88
- Thai Salmon and Carrot Salad   90
- Warm Kale Quinoa Salad   92
- Sweet Potato Buddha Bowl with Chickpeas   94
- Spinach Quiche (Without the Crust)   96
- Lemon Chicken Avocado Salad   98
- Creamy Kabocha Squash and Roasted Red Pepper Pasta   100

DELICIOUS MEALS UNDER 500 CALORIES FOR FASTING DAYS   103

- Slow-Cooked Seafood Ramen   104
- Ginger Maple Glazed Salmon   106
- Caprese Zoodles   108
- Meatball and Tomato Soup   110
- Lentil Soup   112
- Lemon Garlic Butter Chicken with Green Beans Skillet   114

Honey Mustard Pork Chops	116
Spicy Chicken and Avocado Wrap	118
Shrimp and Broccoli	120
Delicious Veggie and Hummus Sandwich	122
Roast Chicken and Sweet Potatoes	124
Lamb Chops with Wild Rice and Quinoa	126
Butter Baked Salmon and Asparagus	128
Gnocchi Skillet with Chicken Sausage and Tomatoes	130
Fettucini Carbonara with Green Beans	132
Sesame Chicken	134
Skillet Chipotle Chicken Enchilada Bake	136
Steak and Broccoli Protein Pot	138
Quick Peanut Noodles	140
Cod with Cucumber, Avocado, and Mango Salsa Salad	142
Tuna Nicoise Protein Pot	144
Orecchiette with Pea Pesto and Walnuts	146
Lemon Chicken Kebabs with Tomato and Parsley Salad	148
Fennel Roasted Chicken and Peppers	150
Low-Calorie Chicken Marsala	152
Chicken Burger with Sun-Dried Tomato	154

Conclusion 157
    So, What Next? 158

References 161

BEFORE YOU START READING

As a special gift, I included a logbook and a cookbook with a variety of recipes to suit all tastes and lifestyles and the best part is, you get access to all of them for free.

What's in it for me?

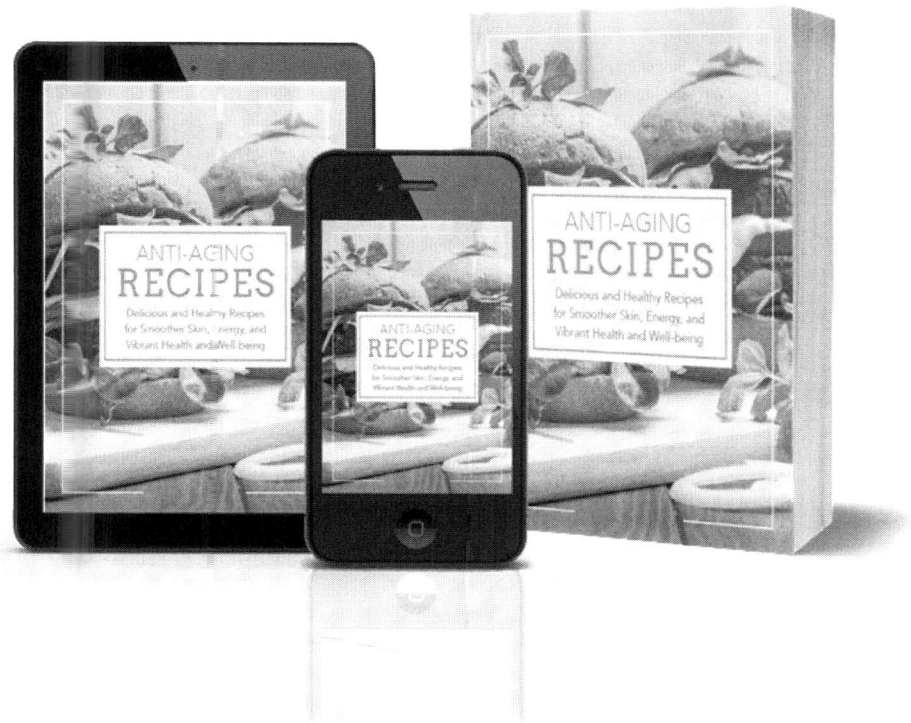

- This cookbook is designed to strengthen your immune system, increase your energy and keep you feeling healthy well into your golden years.
- Recipes to help ensure that the aging process will be gentle and healthful.

- Workout Logbook to help you keep track of your accomplishments and progress
- Log your progress to give you the edge you need to accomplish your goals.

Scan the QR Code

INTRODUCTION

Resilience—this is the word that comes to mind when I think of a woman. We go through childbirth and menstruation as if it's a walk in the park, taking each step in our womanly stride. Yet, why is it that weight gain inevitably creeps upon us as the years progress, with seemingly little control? This is a question that many women, including myself, have pondered for hundreds of years—and the jury is still out on whether there's a clear-cut answer. What we do know for sure is that as women age, their metabolism gradually slows down due to a decrease in lean muscle and an increase in fat. Rapid fluctuations in hormones play a significant role for older women, especially when menopause comes knocking on the door. All these factors result in stubborn body fat refusing to budge no matter how much you diet or hit the gym; so, what can be done about this *travesty*?

There's a new diet trend that has taken the world by storm due to the fact that it doesn't restrict your choices of food while offering a host of impressive health benefits. Sounds too good to be true? Well, surprisingly not! This pattern of eating is known as intermittent fasting (IF) and has been shown to boost metabolism, improve mental clarity, manage neurodegenerative diseases, and even prevent cancer (to name a few)! IF can also help to prevent nerve, joint, and muscle degeneration which is common in women over the age of 50, making it a tempting option for women in this age group ("What to Know About Intermittent Fasting for Women After 50," 2021). The great thing about intermittent fasting is that it's more than just another diet fad—it's a lifestyle! It can easily be adapted into anyone's schedule as you only need to focus on *when* you eat rather than *what* you eat.

Despite the fact that there are several variations of intermittent fasting, there are certain methods that appear to work better than others. For example, fasting according to your circadian rhythms (or body clock) appears to have the best results. So, what exactly does this mean? Essentially, your circadian rhythm is your body's way of tuning into your environment to sync with the timing of meals and exposure to light. When you fast during the evenings and eat during the day, you will aim to eat within a 12-hour eating window and fast for the remaining 12 during the evenings. Not only is this method effective, but it's incredibly straightforward and easy to follow!

If you're wondering what this would look like in your daily routine, you could set your eating window from 8:00 a.m. until 8:00 p.m. every day. This means you're eating all your calories within a 12-hour timeframe and fasting for the remaining 12 while you sleep.

One study conducted in 2016 by PMC labs found that alternating between periods of fasting during the night and eating during daylight hours results in a process known as metabolic switching, whereby the body uses ketones for energy instead of glucose; thus, resulting in weight loss (Longo & Panda, 2016). I'll explain this in deeper detail further in the book, but for now, you need to know the scientific facts.

Essentially, metabolic switching is part of human evolution. In other words, the survivors who endured longer periods without food went on to reproduce, meaning that humans evolved to thrive in a fasted state. During this time, glycogen stores in the liver are depleted as well as fatty acids from cells. In a nutshell, this means your body is burning more fat for fuel, resulting in weight loss. Mark Mattson, a professor of neuroscience at the Johns Hopkins University School of Medicine, claims that exercise can help to speed up this process, which can also help to clear out damaged cells and replace them with newer, healthier ones ("Metabolic Switching May be the Key to Weight Loss and Good Health," 2020).

Another study conducted in 2014 involving humans, found that fasting does in fact combat obesity, asthma, and high blood pressure, as well as rheumatoid arthritis (RA). In the same study, they found that fasting rodents experienced greater protection from cancer, neurodegeneration, and heart disease (Longo & Mattson, 2014). In terms of humans, recent studies have shown that fasting is able to reduce some of the unpleasant side effects of chemotherapy by reducing exposure to toxicity (de Groot et al., 2019). While there is still a lot of research that needs to be done, scientists are feeling positive and excited about their current findings.

If the above findings arouse a feeling of excitement within you, then you're probably dying to get started on your fasting journey! Intermittent fasting can seem daunting—especially if you don't know much about how it works—but with the right know-how and guidance, you'll be a pro in no time at all. This book is designed to provide you with expert, in-depth knowledge about intermittent fasting, as well as a step-by-step guide on how you can personalize IF to your lifestyle. By the time you've finished this book, you'll know all the right foods to eat, when to eat them, and how often to get the best results. When IF is done properly, I can guarantee you that you will see incredible improvements, in both your health and your weight.

The only regret that I have about trying intermittent fasting is not starting it sooner. The good news is that it's never too late to change your lifestyle for the better, so why not start now?

Thank you so much for downloading my book. I would love to hear your thoughts so be sure to leave a review on Amazon. This will help many other people who are in the same situation as you find my book. It would mean a lot to me.

Scan the QR code to leave a Review:

Are you ready? Let's get your fitness education and training started!

CHAPTER 1

UNDERSTANDING INTERMITTENT FASTING

*I*ntermittent fasting is one of the most effective life hacks that you can utilize to boost your metabolism, energy levels, and prevent disease. That said, in order for you to benefit from what IF has to offer, you'll need a clearer understanding of how it works. Before I dive into deeper detail, I'm going to start by explaining more about the history behind intermittent fasting so that you can understand the main ideas, then I'll move on to the intricacies of how it works and why. With all this in mind, let's start with the basics!

The History Behind Intermittent Fasting

Despite what many people think, IF is a perfectly natural phenomenon that has been around for thousands of years. That said, humans aren't the only ones who practice IF; animals do it regularly too, to preserve their health when they're sick. Humans have fasted for a variety of reasons, namely due to religion, or food scarcity (Heffernan, 2020). Thousands of years ago, humans didn't have access to a constant supply of food, meaning that they had to hunt for it. They would often go several hours and even days without food, yet they were still able to function and survive.

Fasting is practiced by nearly every religion in existence, including Christians, Buddhists, Muslims, and Hindus. They see fasting as a way to cleanse and purify the soul, which coincides with what the ancient Greeks believed. Fasting is considered to be one of the most ancient healing practices in the world, with famous world Greek thinkers such as Aristotle and Plato widely advocating its effectiveness. Fasting was also prescribed by Hippocrates of Cos, who was a well-known Greek scientist. The ancient Greeks believed that fasting can be used to cure a wide variety of illnesses, as it allows the body to regenerate and heal. Interestingly, they also believed that fasting promotes cognitive abilities by boosting awareness and mental clarity (Heffernan, 2020).

The notion behind this is that the body naturally increases alertness as a survival mechanism when in a fasted state, to ensure the individual has the mental clarity and energy to hunt for food. Once the individual has satisfied their hunger, the brain can return to a more relaxed state of mind. This is because all types of bodily processes are altered after longer periods of abstaining from food, including: hormones, cellular repair, and genes, which all play factors in how the body functions (Gunnars, 2017). For example, have you ever noticed how you feel after a really big three-course meal on Christmas Day? Your stomach is incredibly full so your mind no longer needs to worry about acquiring food, causing you to feel sluggish and ready for a very long nap!

What is Intermittent Fasting and How Does it Work?

By now, you likely have an idea of what intermittent fasting is, but there's a lot more to it than you originally thought. As I mentioned earlier, intermittent fasting focuses on when you eat rather than what you eat, and involves alternating between cycles of eating and fasting (Gunnars, 2017). This means that you need to consume all your daily calories within your specified eating window, which does involve some planning and restraint. It's important to remember that you cannot consume anything during your fasting period, except for zero or low-calorie drinks such as black coffee, water, herbal tea, or diluted apple cider vinegar. Many people make the mistake of adding sugar and milk to their coffee; therefore, unknowingly breaking their fast.

There are various methods of IF, but the easiest and most common methods are overnight fasting and the 16/8 method. Regardless of which method you choose, the end goal remains the same—to burn fat at a faster pace by revving up your metabolism. Intermittent fasting is widely backed by Mark Mattson, a well-known neuroscientist who spent 25 years of his career studying the science of intermittent fasting. Mattson believes that humans have evolved to withstand long periods without food, to such an extent that they thrive rather than suffer. He also believes that obesity in the modern era is a result of people fasting less and eating more, as food is increasingly more readily available than ever before.

In terms of the mechanisms of IF, I'll explain it as simply as I can. Essentially, intermittent fasting works by inducing a process known as metabolic switching which can be described as the process of the body changing from burning glucose for energy to burning fat instead—which is where the process of weight loss occurs. By fasting, you're increasing the time between the calories burned during your last meal and the next, allowing your body to cut into those stubborn fat stores ("Intermittent Fasting: What is it, and How Does it Work," 2021). One of the main reasons that many people battle to lose weight is because they are constantly eating, providing their bodies with a never-ending source of glucose. As a result, the body is unable to burn through fat stores preventing you from losing weight. The great thing about intermittent fasting is that it ensures that you're giving your body the chance to burn that extra fat when you otherwise wouldn't.

Why Choose Intermittent Fasting Over Traditional Diets?

Many women have wondered why they should opt for IF when they could simply practice a calorie-restricted diet instead. Keeping slim and healthy is something that every individual strives for meaning that it's important to choose a weight loss option that is safe and effective, with the most added benefits. That said, the comparison between IF and basic calorie restriction has always been a hot debate, which is why I'm going to address it for you now. When it comes to this, I always like to look at the scientific evidence to draw a conclusion.

Intermittent Fasting vs. Calorie Restriction

Essentially, calorie-restricting diets involve reducing the total number of daily calories you consume. For example, if you typically eat 2000 calories per day, you would aim to consume between 300-500 fewer calories to shed some pounds. The idea behind this is that your body will naturally lose weight by providing it with less energy—which is correct Intermittent fasting on the other hand, focuses more on weekly calorie averages than daily calorie averages. With calorie restriction, you're able to eat food whenever you please, as long as you're not exceeding your daily calorie count (William, 2021). IF; however, restricts your hours between fasting and non-fasting, which can take a lot more self-control—but this depends *entirely* on the individual—which brings me to my next point.

An in-depth experiment was conducted by the University of Illinois whereby they compared calorie restriction with alternate-day fasting. In a nutshell, alternate-day fasting involves alternating between fasting days and feasting days. On the fasting days, you are only permitted to consume 25% of your typical daily calories. This experiment was conducted for one year and included a wide variety of 100 participants who were all screened for their BMI and pregnancy status. Their age range fell between 18-65 with BMIs ranging from 25 to 39.9 (moderate to severely overweight). They were split into three groups, with one group fasting, the other group restricting calories, and the third group having no control whatsoever. In terms of weight loss, the alternate-day fasting group and the calorie-restriction group lost almost the same amount of weight, meaning no diet is necessarily better than the other (William, 2021). So, what does this mean?

Essentially, it is entirely up to the individual! You need to decide on a method that works best for you and your lifestyle. You just need to remember that calorie-restricted diets involve a lot of planning and tracking of meals, compared to IF where you simply need to skip a meal and eat what you like once your eating window arrives. You also need to take into account the benefits of each type of diet, as this should ultimately be your deciding factor. And, most importantly, intermittent fasting has one advantage over every other type of diet—*it's not a diet*. The one problem with diets is that they're difficult to stick to and maintain, and you'll likely end up gaining back all the weight you initially lost. With IF, you can implement the plan into your lifestyle until you don't even notice you're doing it! Plus, IF has a host of unique benefits that most traditional diets lack (I'll dive into deeper detail later).

For now, you're probably wondering exactly how fasting will affect certain groups of people, specifically women over the age of 50. This is an important question that many women have asked and needs to be addressed thoroughly and accurately, so let's get started.

Intermittent Fasting and Women Over 50

Losing weight when you're over the age of 50 is a long, hard, uphill battle that many women can relate to. As we grow older, aching muscles, sleep problems, muscle loss, and a slowed metabolism all contribute to weight gain. As a result, our self-esteem takes a hit and we tend to lose all hope of regaining our confidence and health. On top of this, older women are more prone to illnesses such as cancer and musculoskeletal disorders, and these effects can be devastating. So, is intermittent fasting a viable solution to these risks? Some people claim that IF is the equivalent of the fountain of youth for older women, by preventing disease and burning fat—but just how true is this? Well, you're about to find out!

According to Nair & Khawale (2016), cancer is one of the leading causes of death worldwide, and this is especially true for older women. Five of the most common cancers found in women are breast, cervix, lung, colorectum, and stomach. The good news is that fasting is a proven prognostic tool used to fight against diseases such as cancer, as it can stop the progression of the disease and make the cancer cells more sensitive to cancer treatment such as radiotherapy and chemotherapy.

More recent studies have found that fasting stops the growth of tumors by a process of angiogenesis. Because of this process, the tumor cannot grow due to a lack of blood supply caused by fasting, as tumors can only grow as large as 0.5 mm without sufficient blood supply (Nair & Khawale, 2016). Similar results have been found in mice, where the growth of tumors was also suppressed by the introduction of fasting. This is why older women in particular can benefit from IF, as it not only helps reduce calories but also shows significant promise in fighting symptoms of cancer and aiding treatment. Intermittent fasting also naturally reduces the total number of calories you consume, meaning that you'll likely lose weight. The idea behind weight loss is simple—as long as you're burning more calories than you consume you'll drop the extra pounds. As we grow older and menopause comes into play, it may be necessary to make an extra effort to help your body burn more calories, which is where IF comes in.

One 2017 study found that people who consumed their daily calories within a four-hour window consumed 650 fewer total calories than those who did not. For postmenopausal women, research has shown that IF is particularly beneficial for weight maintenance and control; yet another study found that fasting for a period of 36-hours results in a decrease of 1900 total daily calories, even if they ate more calories during their next eating window. According to Kim et al. (2017), fasting for 16 weeks without any calorie tracking whatsoever can significantly fight obesity as well as a variety of other metabolic disorders. In fact, benefits can begin to show after only six weeks, according to the very same study.

While the above information is only the tip of the iceberg when it comes to IF in older women, there are so many myths surrounding intermittent fasting! There are a ton of rumors doing the rounds on IF that need to be debunked, so keep reading to find out exactly what they are and why they aren't true. Let's dive in!

7 Myths About Intermittent Fasting: Debunked!

Now that you're all clued up on some of the most interesting facts about IF, it's time to educate yourself on the things that are simply *not true* about this pattern of eating! I'm sure you've probably heard people saying that "IF eats away at your muscle and slows down your metabolism." Well, there's absolutely zero scientific evidence to back this up, and far more evidence to support the exact *opposite* of these claims! While these are some of the most common myths, below I'm going to cover some less conventional ones that may surprise you.

Skipping Breakfast is Bad for You

One of the most common phrases that you've likely heard is that "breakfast is the most important meal of the day." But exactly how accurate is this? Well, according to most studies, this is not accurate at all. Many people believe that skipping breakfast will result in intense cravings leading to overeating later on in the day, while others believe that skipping breakfast is bad for the brain and energy levels. As we've already uncovered, fasting is good for mental sharpness and alertness; you're better off giving breakfast a miss if you're not hungry (Gunnars, 2019).

In a study conducted in 2016, it was discovered that adults who consumed breakfast weighed the same as those who did not. This study contained a large group of overweight individuals and was done in a controlled environment. This shows that breakfast doesn't seem to have much of an effect on your weight, as long as you listen to your body's signals (Dhurandhar et al., 2014). If you find you are starving in the mornings, then you can adjust your schedule to include breakfast and fast later on in the day. If not, then don't feel obliged to eat breakfast if you're not hungry, rather listen to your body's hunger signals instead of eating for the sake of it.

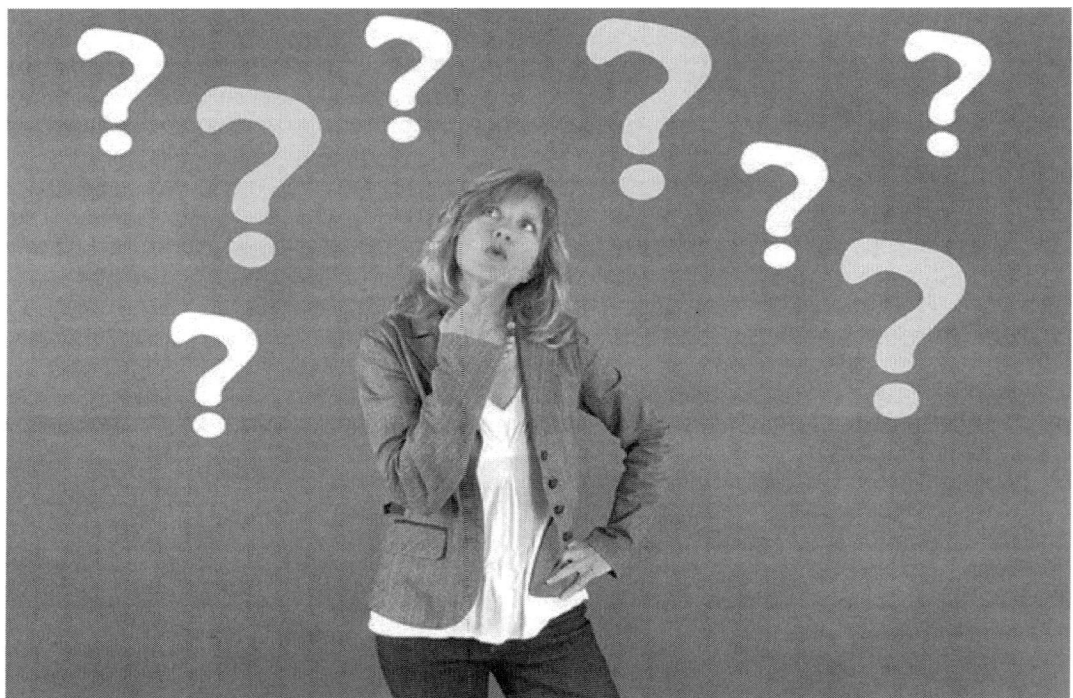

If you think about it, skipping breakfast and eating your first meal at around noon can save you an extra 300-400 calories, which could be the difference between you gaining or losing weight.

Fasting Causes Your Body to Hit Starvation Mode

Many anti-fasters will argue that fasting causes your body to enter a state of starvation; therefore, slowing down your rate of fat burning and storing fat. While this may be true for very extended periods of fasting, anywhere from eight to 48 hours of fasting will boost your metabolism rather than slow it down. Long-term weight loss can result in your body burning fewer calories over time, but it's important to remember that this isn't exclusively true for IF alone—this will happen with any eating pattern that results in weight loss over time. This is why many people reach a plateau once they lose a significant amount of weight, as the body's metabolism naturally slows down as a survival mechanism which makes it harder to maintain their current weight or lose more (Gunnars, 2019).

Essentially, you should be doing daily short-term fasts to boost your metabolism and reap the full benefits. Studies have shown fasting for anywhere up to 48 hours can boost your metabolism by a whopping 3.6%-14% (Gunnars, 2019). As long as you're not starving yourself for weeks on end, your metabolism will be perfectly fine.

Fasting Leads to Overeating

Some people believe that fasting will only lead to overeating once the fast is over and the eating window begins. While it's true that you'll naturally be hungry after a longer fast, it's unlikely that you'll overcompensate to such an extent that you gain the calories you forfeited during your fast. For example, if you have an eating window of only six hours and a fasting period of eighteen hours, it's highly unlikely that you'll manage to consume enough excess calories in those six hours to compensate for eighteen hours without food.

Not to mention that your insulin levels will naturally be lowered from the fast, as well as giving other hormones the boost that encourages fat loss naturally. If you need some scientific backing, then you'll be interested to know that a 2002 study discovered that a 24-hour fast only leads to the consumption of an extra 500 calories the following day, which doesn't even begin to compare with the 2400 calorie loss from the 24-hour fast (Johnstone et al., 2002).

Fasting is Unhealthy

Fasting has been shown to promote longevity through altering the expression of genes, with animal studies showing a definitive lengthening of their lifespan. Fasting is also healthy for the immune system and the brain, and also fights inflammation, heart disease, and oxidative stress (Gunnars, 2019).

Eating Often Boosts Metabolism

I'm sure you've heard people say that eating lots of small meals throughout the day is a metabolism-booster; while there's nothing wrong with doing this, it's certainly inaccurate to believe that you're increasing your metabolism and burning more calories. The truth is, the total number of calories that you consume in one day combined with periods of fasting will increase your metabolism, not the number of meals you eat. While it's true that the digestion of food does burn calories (approximately 10% of your total calories for the day), the number will remain the same regardless of how many portions you consume them in (Gunnars, 2019).

For example, let's say that your daily calorie requirement to lose weight is 1500 calories. Regardless of whether you split this into three portions of 500 calories or seven portions of 200 calories, you'll still burn the same number of calories. One review of several studies that were conducted in 1997 showed that there is no correlation between meal frequency and energy balance, concluding that body weight and metabolism are likely influenced by total daily food intake (Bellisle et al., 1997).

You Will Experience Brain Fog

Have you ever heard of the term gluconeogenesis? Essentially, this process occurs when glucose, lipids, or protein are broken down in the liver, brain, and kidneys as sources of energy. It was initially believed that this process only occurred in the liver and kidneys, but now we know it takes place in the brain too. That said, this is the reason why this myth is simply not true! Some people believe that refraining from eating carbohydrates will result in the brain malfunctioning or experiencing brain fog. While it's perfectly normal to feel a little bit shaky or dizzy in the initial stages of a fast, your brain certainly won't shut down!

It is assumed that the brain needs a constant supply of glucose to function; however, the brain can do this itself through the process of gluconeogenesis. The liver is also able to produce ketones to function, which will be discussed in the next chapter. Ketones are produced after long periods of fasting and are used for energy in place of glucose when the body runs out of supplies. These ketones provide the brain with all the fuel that it needs to function optimally without the need for a continuous flow of food. This process is known as ketosis (Gunnars, 2019).

Fasting Results in Muscle Loss

This is one of the biggest myths surrounding IF! This fact isn't true for a multitude of reasons, but what you need to know is that fasting is better for muscle growth and preservation than regular calorie restriction. This is why bodybuilders practice IF with many of them consuming only one large meal at the end of the day, this plan is known as the "Warrior Diet." One study conducted in 2007 found that people who consumed one large meal in the evening and fasted during the day showed a significant increase in muscle mass (Stote et al., 2007).

Another 2011 study aimed to compare intermittent fasting with calorie restriction, where the main focus was on weight loss and muscle. The results indicated that both groups lost a similar amount of weight, but the people who fasted lost the least muscle mass (Varady, 2011). These results are only two of the many studies on this, so it's safe to say that this myth is busted!

CHAPTER 2

THE MANY BENEFITS OF INTERMITTENT FASTING

As you've learned, intermittent fasting boasts some truly impressive benefits that I'm sure you're dying to know more about. In this chapter, you'll learn the scientific facts behind each benefit, as well as exactly how the process works and why. By the end of this section, there should be no benefit-based question unanswered!

How Intermittent Fasting Helps You Lose Weight

Intermittent fasting helps to facilitate weight loss via several fascinating mechanisms. Let's dive in!

Intermittent Fasting Decreases Leptin and Insulin Levels

When you fast, several bodily processes change as a response to the lack of food, including your insulin and leptin levels among various other genes and hormones. If you're wondering what leptin means for your body, it's essentially your hunger hormone that signals your body when you're feeling full. Fasting results in your insulin and leptin levels dropping, which is exactly what you want to happen if you're looking to burn fat. It was initially believed that only a drop in insulin was required for fat burning to occur, but more recent studies have found that both insulin and leptin need to drop in order to be successful.

Insulin on the other hand, removes glucose stores from the bloodstream; thus, lowering blood sugar levels. It does this by removing glucose from the blood and sending it to nearby cells which burn the glucose into fuel for energy or store it as fat—not ideal. When insulin levels are too high, they prevent the body from burning fat stores for energy, which is why lowered insulin levels are ideal for weight loss. Researchers from Yale tested the effects of insulin and leptin on rats when fasting, and they discovered that when the two are lowered together, the rats experienced a significantly higher rate of fat burning as glucose was turned into ketones for fuel ("Drop in Both Insulin and Leptin Needed for Fat Burning to Occur—Diabetes," 2018).

Additional studies have found that IF resulted in a 3%-8% reduction in weight for overweight and obese men and women over 3-24 weeks, with a concurrent reduction in waist circumference of 3%-7% during the same time. In another 2018 study looking at overweight adults, researchers discovered that groups of individuals who fasted also experienced an average weight loss of 15 pounds over a timeframe of 3-12 months (Coyle, 2018).

When it comes to women in particular, there are limited studies that show how IF can be an effective weight-loss method. Two of these studies involved the comparison of a typical calorie-restricted diet and the 5:2 method of IF. For this method, the participants fasted for two days of the week and resumed normal eating for the remaining five days. The calorie-restricted group were told to cut their normal daily calories by 25%, while the fasting group only had to fast two days of the week (Wallis, 2021).

In terms of the results, both groups of 100 women lost the same amount of weight over the six month period, but there was one critical difference—the fasting group had far superior blood sugar levels and a much larger reduction in actual fat loss. This is likely due to how fasting initiates the fat-burning process of ketosis. This is further backed by another 2019 study conducted by Varady, a well-known doctor and researcher on fasting. They found that alternate-day fasting—another form of IF—produced the most significant reduction in insulin levels. IF was more than twice as efficient at improving the body's response to insulin than simply cutting calories alone (Wallis, 2021).

Keeping that in mind, I do need to mention that scientists are still exploring how IF affects weight loss—in women in particular—over longer periods of time. What we do know is that IF is an effective method for weight loss over short periods. The good news is that there are certain methods of fasting that appear to work better for older women in particular.

Intermittent Fasting and Heart Health

As we grow older, we become more susceptible to conditions such as high cholesterol, high triglyceride concentrations, and hypertension. All these factors combined can contribute to heart disease, which can be seriously life-threatening. So, to prevent heart disease from becoming a threat, it's a good idea to maintain a lifestyle that promotes healthy eating patterns. That said, intermittent fasting has the potential to manage symptoms associated with these conditions.

Researchers have conducted studies with both men and women who are at risk for heart disease due to being significantly overweight with high blood pressure, high triglycerides, and cholesterol. The researchers wanted to find out whether fasting would help with these symptoms, so they introduced it to different groups. After only 8 weeks the researchers found that the 16 men and women both showed a decrease in hypertension by 6%, and their LDL cholesterol and triglycerides were lowered by 25% and 32% respectively.

One important fact that I must mention is that researchers are still looking for a stronger link between fasting and the above, as some of the findings were not as consistent as they would ideally prefer. That said, hopefully, as time and technology progress, scientists will be able to find a more definitive answer to this question. For now, we can only anticipate some exciting new revelations, as the current studies are certainly promising!

Intermittent Fasting and the Brain

Before writing this section, I came across a truly fascinating article on the incredible benefits that fasting can have on the brain. Initially, I thought it sounded too good to be true until I saw who backed the information—none other than neurosurgeon Dr. Rahul Jandial, author of *Neurofitness* whereby he explains in detail why IF is so beneficial for brain functioning. As I mentioned in the previous chapter, fasting has been around for hundreds of years as a way to cleanse the mind, body, and soul, and Dr. Jandial believes they have good reason to do so.

Intermittent fasting benefits the brain in several ways; for example, fasting causes the body to release more Human Growth Hormone (HGH) which naturally reduces inflammation in the body and induces a process called autophagy. Part of this process; however, includes the release of more brain-derived neurotrophic factor (BDNF), which influences how your brain functions. All these functions combined result in the preservation and regeneration of brain cells, reducing inflammation while getting rid of waste in the cells.

The reason why this happens is because of our natural survival instinct. In prehistoric times, the brain had to produce specific hormones during times of survival and self-preservation. Evolution has pre-programmed human beings to perform at their best when food is scarce and the body perceives a threat, meaning that neuroplasticity of the brain and resistance to disease is at their absolute peak during metabolic switching. In simpler terms, when there is less glucose in the body and more ketones due to no food, the body ramps up its cognitive abilities and boosts immunity from disease as a sophisticated survival mechanism.

One of the benefits that make IF trump calorie restriction is connected with brain function, and I'll explain why. Calorie restriction, as the name suggests, means you're quite literally restricting your calories to a significantly lower number than you're accustomed to. If you typically consume 1,400 calories per day and you're at a plateau, then you may decide to restrict your calories to 1,000 per day. This means that you'll be constantly hungry throughout the day, which isn't ideal. With IF, you might feel hungry for intermittent periods but this is so that your body can burn through its fat reserves.

How often you do this depends entirely on the method that you choose, but you're burning fat nevertheless. The best way to combat hunger is by filling up on water and low-calorie tea and coffee, as well as reminding yourself why you are fasting and the benefits you will reap if you persevere. Keeping busy also helps, as this prevents you from fixating on food when you don't have anything else to do.

In terms of benefits for your brain, the switch from glucose to ketones is the exhaust for your brain. This process keeps it working at an optimal level by growing connections between neurons, boosting overall cognition, and preventing neurodegeneration—all in the name of survival! The brain truly is an incredible thing.

Intermittent Fasting and Alzheimer's

Alzheimer's is one of the most common neurodegenerative disorders, with no cure currently on the horizon. Alzheimer's is not only traumatic for the patient, but for their loved ones too. That said, when it comes to this devastating disease, the best possible cure is prevention. While there is still more research that needs to be conducted in humans, there is some very promising research in animals indicating a positive relationship between fasting and the prevention of Alzheimer's (Gunnars, 2021).

Several studies in rodents have found that the introduction of fasting reduced the severity of Alzheimer's and delayed the inception of the disease. In fact, additional studies on animals have found that fasting can help prevent other neurodegenerative conditions such as Huntington's and Parkinson's disease (Gunnars, 2021).

In terms of humans, there is some positive evidence. A study was conducted on patients with Alzheimer's who were asked to fast every night for 12 hours, while the doctors closely examined their symptoms before and after they began fasting. Out of the participants, an impressive 90% of them noticed significant improvements in their symptoms, which is really promising (Bredesen, 2014).

How Does Fasting Boost Cognitive Functioning in Mice?

Brain-derived neurotrophic factor (BDNF) is a chemical present in all mammals. Not only does it make the brain more resistant to stress, but it also promotes learning, memory, and the production of new nerve cells in the hippocampus—the part of the brain that stores memory.

Studies have found that mice also experience growth and regeneration in brain cells when they are exposed to a fasting regime. Their brains enter a resource preservation mode whereby cell growth is turned off and dysfunctional cells are removed. Once the mice resume eating again, the cells and proteins begin to grow and generate new synapses. (Wnuk, 2018). Who would have thought we have so much in common with rodents?

How to Fast for Brain Power

According to doctors, you don't need to fast every single day to reap the brain-boosting benefits of fasting. In fact, fasting as little as twice per week is enough to enjoy all the brain-enhancing benefits with very little sacrifice! According to Dr. Jandial (2020), he fasts twice weekly with each fast lasting 16-hours. During these two days, he skips breakfast and lunch and only eats dinner with his family. He doesn't fuss over what's for dinner, he'll just have whatever his wife and kids have; because he's fasted for the entire day, he can pretty much enjoy whatever he likes without worrying about over-eating—the beauty of intermittent fasting!

Another effective way to do this is to simply skip breakfast most days, which is pretty easy, especially if you have a busy schedule. While it may take your body a few days to adapt, you'll find that you very rarely feel hungry before noon and you'll be full of energy. Remember, there is absolutely *zero* scientific evidence that supports breakfast as the most important meal of the day.

While there's nothing wrong with enjoying the occasional breakfast on the weekend or a special outing, there's no reason to force it every morning. Dr. Jandial also refrains from late-night snacking, as this is where most of the damage is done. While it's okay to slip up occasionally, try not to make a habit of it or you'll ruin all your hard work.

Who Shouldn't Fast?

One of the most important things you need to consider before fasting is whether or not it's safe. While IF is an awesome lifestyle hack and is generally safe for most people, there are certain groups of people who should approach it with caution. Below I'm going to list the groups of people who should avoid fasting in the interests of their safety.

According to Buckingham (2020), these are the groups of people who should think twice:

You Really, Really Love Eating

If you are the type of person who simply loves to eat, then you may really struggle with IF. Fasting takes a tremendous amount of self-control and perseverance: meaning you really need to *want* to fast and enjoy the benefits. If you feel that you're not in the right mindset to start fasting, then you may want to wait until you are ready. The reason being, not having the right mindset can cause you to form an unhealthy obsession over food where you're constantly fantasizing about eating despite knowing you can't. When this happens, you may find yourself binging on foods when you usually wouldn't due to intense hunger and cravings.

Remember, every person is different, so it's important to find a pattern of eating that suits your lifestyle. If not, you'll only make yourself miserable and won't succeed in your endeavors. Do what makes *you* comfortable.

You Have a Very Demanding Job

While it's true that some people are able to perform high-energy jobs without any sustenance, others may struggle. I know people who can easily power through the workday with nothing more than coffee and water, whereas others can't make it past eight a.m. So, this depends entirely on how comfortable you feel. That said, if you are someone who regularly feels the need to eat and you have a high-focus, high-energy job, you may want to consider another method for weight loss. For example, if you are a construction worker, an Olympic athlete, or a surgeon, then it may not be the best idea to abstain from food for long periods.

You Have a History of Eating Disorders

Since many individuals with eating disorders tend to obsess over when they eat, how they eat, and what they eat, fasting is not something that should be encouraged in any way. Any pattern of eating that includes the restriction of food can trigger negative behavior in someone with this kind of history. If you've previously battled one and have recovered, you should sit down with your therapist and discuss the safety and viability of IF. Remember, you should always prioritize your mental health!

You Battle to Sleep

While it's a good idea to avoid eating too much too late in the evenings, ending your eating window too early in the day can also pose some issues. For example, eating too early can result in you feeling hungry before bed, and this will only make it harder to refrain from late-night snacking. A good night's rest is absolutely crucial for maintaining a healthy mind and body; those who are sleep-deprived often face a myriad of health complications over time. During sleep, your body regenerates any damaged tissue and consolidates important information, which can be compromised if you're not sleeping well. So, you're probably wondering exactly how fasting influences this.

Well, earlier I mentioned how fasting makes your brain more alert; if you schedule your fast too close to bedtime, you may find it difficult to sleep as your body is on high alert. Another reason for disrupted sleep is low blood sugar levels, as this can cause you to wake up in the middle of the night feeling anxious and unable to fall back to sleep easily. When you wake up in the middle of the night too often, you disrupt your sleep cycle, which result in you missing out on REM sleep—vital for memory retention and learning.

To combat these problems, it's always best to make sure that your eating window ends no more than four hours before you plan to go to sleep. There's nothing worse than going to bed with a growling stomach, and you'll wake up feeling extra hungry and tempted to overeat, which isn't making things any easier.

You're Pregnant or Breastfeeding

While this should be fairly obvious for us women, it's still important to mention. In order for a woman to carry a healthy child and produce sufficient milk, she needs to eat a variety of foods throughout the day. When you're fasting, you're likely going to lose weight which shouldn't be your primary goal while pregnant or breastfeeding. The same goes for women trying for a baby—you don't want to lose too much weight too quickly while trying to conceive, as this may disrupt your monthly cycle. As we know, fasting does influence the metabolism, and may even disrupt menstruation and fertility in severe cases.

You Have Digestive Problems

If you regularly suffer from digestive problems, you may want to consult your doctor before trying IF. The reason being, some people report experiencing changes in their stomach during the initial stages of IF, and these may worsen if you already experience problems. In addition to this, extended fasts typically require a relatively large meal once the eating window begins, which may cause digestive upset for sensitive stomachs.

While not the most common, some people have reported bloating, indigestion, and constipation in the initial stages of fasting. If these side effects aren't for you, then practice with caution!

You Have Diabetes

If you, or someone you love has diabetes then you'll know how scary a low blood sugar episode can be. Sweating, shaking, nausea, and weakness are all par for the course, and you certainly don't want to bring this on. As you know, fasting does have an effect on glucose and insulin levels, so if you're already on medication to regulate diabetes it's not a good idea to throw fasting into the mix. For example, if you have type 1 diabetes, you'll know that your body struggles to produce insulin. This means you have to inject insulin throughout the day to ensure that you don't enter a life-threatening state known as hyperglycemia (too much sugar in the blood). With fasting, you're likely to lower already dangerous levels of insulin which can have devastating results.

If you really want to try IF, it's highly advisable to first consult with your doctor. If you don't, you may find yourself in some unsafe situations where your medication and the fasting clash, which can have really dangerous consequences.

You're on Medication That Requires Food

If you're on chronic medications you'll likely find that they need to be taken with some food rather than on an empty stomach. Many vitamins also require a meal in order to ensure that they are optimally absorbed by the body—iron in particular. Iron supplements are notorious for causing nausea when taken on an empty stomach, and those with iron deficiency need to ensure they are taking their dose regularly. When you take certain medications without food, you may find yourself experiencing some unpleasant side effects such as nausea, dizziness, or light-headedness. While you may be able to work around the timing of your medication and fast, this may prove a little tricky if your medication needs to be taken at a very specific time.

You Work Erratic Hours

The great thing about IF is that you are able to adjust the method according to what best suits your lifestyle. That said, some lifestyles simply cannot accommodate IF without compromising your health in some way. For example, if you are a security officer who works the nightshift and your job requires a significant amount of movement, you may struggle to get through your fast. This is especially true if your shifts often change from day to night, as you'll struggle to find a set routine for your fasting and sleeping schedules. You may also experience some undesirable side effects during the beginning of your fast, which may negatively affect your job performance if you're forced to align your fast with busy working hours.

You Have a Very Intense Workout Regime

While it is still possible to gain muscle while fasting, you'll need to make sure that your eating window and workout times coincide. If you follow a heavy exercise routine that includes heavy weight-lifting, marathons, or CrossFit, you're not going to cope with the pressure without sufficient fuel. In order to get the most out of your workout, you'll need to make sure you're eating some complex carbs beforehand and a healthy dose of protein post-workout in order to help your muscles build and repair. When you do a heavy workout, your muscles require glycogen to repair and build, meaning that depriving your body of food for longer periods of time could render your workout pointless.

Ideally, you should be eating a recovery meal approximately 1-2 hours after your training to replenish energy levels, meaning you'll need to make sure that you plan around this when you fast. In other words, don't schedule a heavy workout when you know you will be in your fasting window. For example, if you regularly train then you could try the 5:2 approach. This means that you only fast for two days of the week, so you can use your fasting days to rest, and the remaining five days for training. That said, this is simply one example of how you can schedule your fast to suit your personal needs and you can alter it as you please.

You Have a Life-Threatening Illness

While there are plenty of studies that promote IF as a way to prevent and fight disease, it's always best to speak to your doctor before making any significant lifestyle change. When you are very sick, you need to prioritize your calorie intake and make sure that you are giving your body the vitamins and minerals that it requires to get better. While IF can help to prepare your immune system to better fight disease, it's better to speak to your doctor first—if you are already unwell. If none of the above conditions apply to you, then chances are IF should blend in well with your lifestyle and health goals. If you're still unsure whether IF is the right choice, then you can always consult your doctor to decide which is the best method to safely and effectively change your lifestyle and improve your overall health.

CHAPTER 3

AGING AND INTERMITTENT FASTING FOR OLDER WOMEN

One of the primary reasons (besides weight loss) that interests women in fasting is its supposed effects on anti-aging. The question on many people's lips is whether this is true or not; can the simple act of abstaining from food *really* slow down the aging process and prevent weight gain? As women, we want to try and age as gracefully as possible, but the slower the better! In this chapter, all of these questions will be answered in detail with scientific evidence to help you understand how the process works. This will help you decide for yourself whether fasting truly is the fountain of youth or not. Let's take a closer look.

How Does Aging Hamper Weight Loss in Women?

As women grow older, the diet and exercise routine that used to keep us slim and trim suddenly leaves us 30 pounds heavier! Why is life so cruel and unfair? As women age, the weight we gain has very little to do with what we eat. Sadly, this is because of our changing hormones, aging, lifestyle, and genetics. Since we lose muscle mass at a much faster rate when we're older, our bodies burn fat at a slower rate, resulting in weight gain. Not only does this mess with our self-esteem but it can also be detrimental to our health and wellbeing if left unchecked, which is why it's so important to take control before it's too late.

As we know, intermittent fasting is an excellent way to burn fat at a faster rate and enjoy a host of health benefits such as decreased inflammation, disease prevention, and increased alertness. Some people believe—based on certain animal studies—that IF can act as the fountain of youth and help to prevent aging through various metabolic processes. While this may sound like something out of a science-fiction novel, there is some truth to the fact that IF is associated with aging and cell regeneration, but the jury is still out on the verdict on humans. That said, I'm going to outline below some of the most interesting pieces of information on this topic so that you can decide for yourself!

How Does Fasting Slow the Aging Process?

Before I dive into the nitty-gritty of things, I want to emphasize the fact that most longevity studies on fasting have been conducted on animals. While this is not to say that these benefits don't also apply to humans, there are still more studies that need to be conducted in order to be absolutely certain. That said, IF does help manage and prevent certain neurodegenerative and musculoskeletal conditions that are associated with aging in older adults.

For now, what you need to know is that fasting is also said to play a role in cell regeneration and autophagy in humans. All of the above-mentioned processes contribute to anti-aging, so they're definitely worth taking a closer look at. For now, I'm going to outline some of the most reputable studies on fasting and factors associated with anti-aging—you'll be amazed at some of the findings!

Studies Supporting Fasting and Anti-Aging

If you're anything like me, I have to see something to believe it. Not everything you read online is true unless it's been scientifically backed by verified, reputable studies—which is why I decided to dedicate an entire chapter to this. As we already know, fasting causes glucose levels in the blood to drop, resulting in the body switching from burning glucose, to fat stores for energy. This process is known as ketosis, where there are more ketones in the blood allowing the body to burn fat at an optimal level. When it comes to IF and aging, researchers from Harvard have found a significant association between fasting and an extended lifespan—at least in animals.

According to recent Harvard studies, fasting works by causing the mitochondria in cells to produce more energy at a faster pace, all while remaining in the most youthful state. Speculation from Harvard professors is that the cells are able to work optimally when they are not preoccupied with other processes associated with digesting food, particularly at night ("Is Intermittent Fasting Safe for Older Adults," 2020).

In another study, scientists from the Okinawa Institute of Science and Technology

Graduate University in Japan aimed to find out how fasting affects the appearance of aging skin. This study in particular interested me, as I'm always looking for new ways to enhance the look and feel of my skin (surgery-free, of course)! Essentially, the scientists were looking at the effects of metabolism on the skin and how gluconeogenesis plays an impact. If you need a reminder, gluconeogenesis is when the body extracts glucose from sources such as amino acids instead of carbohydrates as a result of fasting. Part of this process involves an increase in the production of pyrimidine and purines which are known to increase the levels of antioxidants in the body ("Fasting Can Slow Down Aging," 2020).

Antioxidants are well-known for their incredible benefits to health and wellbeing, and this includes youthful, glowing skin. This release of antioxidants, as the researchers found, is a simple way to restore balance while the body is hungry during a fast. As a result, the body is also able to fight common causes of aging such as oxidative stress and harmful free radicals. In order to truly reap the benefits of fasting and healthy skin, you'll need to make sure that you break your fast with a wholesome, healthy meal. If you don't you'll be undoing the effects fasting has on your skin health ("Fasting Can Slow Down Aging, 2020).

In another study published by the International Journal of Environmental Research and Public Health, researchers split a group of 45 women over the age of 60 into two groups—a control group where the women were permitted to eat normally, and the experimental group who were asked to fast for 16-hours. They ate their last meal at 8:00 p.m., and refrained from eating until noon the following day; this group only changed the timing of their eating and not the actual foods that they ate (Eenfeldt, 2020).

The results were positive—the fasting group lost an average of three pounds in body weight and fat mass over the six-week period, whereas the control group who did not fast experienced no weight loss whatsoever. Interestingly, none of the women over 60 who fasted experienced any loss of muscle or any negative side effects. So, what exactly does this tell us about fasting for older women? Well, this study, along with several others mentioned above, all indicate that fasting can be an exceptionally powerful tool for older women (Eenfeldt, 2020).

Fasting and Autophagy Explained

If you've never heard of autophagy before then you are not alone! Another term for autophagy is "self-eating," which is exactly what the cells in our body do during the fasting process. While this may sound like a cause for concern, autophagy is a perfectly healthy process that rejuvenates the cell. In a nutshell, autophagy is a form of cellular repair whereby cells remove excess waste that they no longer need. Our bodies contain an incomprehensible number of cells that build up as we age, and this can result in damaged molecules building up which could become harmful. This process ensures that the body continues to function as it should as all cells are working optimally (otherwise known as homeostasis). This means that damaged molecules are either completely destroyed, or they are recycled into new forms that can be used to repair and rejuvenate damaged cells (Davis, 2021).

By now you're probably wondering what on earth prompts your body to do this, and how it knows when old cells need to be regenerated? Well, as you may have guessed, intermittent fasting can be a trigger for this process and I'll explain why. When the body is stressed, the cells become deprived of essential things such as oxygen and nutrients. Your body acknowledges that something is not right and responds by finding alternative means of providing your body with extra strength while under stress. This stress is caused by a noticeable lack of food through fasting, so the cells in the body have to ramp up performance as a response to this. One of the ways it does this is through autophagy, by clearing out damaged cells and toxins that are hindering the body (Davis, 2021).

According to a 2018 review on the effects of eating patterns on autophagy, there is a significant relationship between fasting, calorie restriction, and the process of autophagy (Bagherniya et al., 2018). That said, it is important to mention that most of the studies that have been carried out have been conducted on animals. While this is not to say that there isn't evidence of this process in humans, animals have been the primary focus. Researchers are still trying to discover whether fasting causes the process of autophagy in the human brain, though animal studies have proven to be promising.

How Long Do You Need to Fast to Reach Autophagy?

This depends heavily on the speed of your metabolism and a few other factors, but the general consensus is that autophagy kicks in properly after two to four days of fasting. In some cases, autophagy has been seen in humans after only 24 hours, but researchers still need to perform more studies in order to better understand exactly how long autophagy truly takes to kick in. That said, fasting for such prolonged periods of time to attain possible benefits doesn't seem wise, so always consult your doctor beforehand and weigh up the benefits and risks (Davis, 2021).

Another issue that arises is the fact that autophagy is extremely difficult to measure. While some studies have tried, measuring autophagy in humans is still a mystery to many researchers. This is because it is very difficult to observe autophagy in action as this process is continuous and requires observations over longer periods of time. This is why scientists study autophagy primarily in animals and cell cultures, which is where most of the current information comes from (RD., 2020).

Should Older Women Rely on Autophagy for Anti-Aging?

Fasting has so many proven positive effects on health that don't include autophagy but can also be linked to anti-aging and improved health. Fasting should instead be utilized in order to improve overall health through weight loss and disease prevention, as this alone will extend your lifespan without the need for autophagy.

So, how can you best go about making the big transition to intermittent fasting?

Tips for Transitioning to Intermittent Fasting Properly

Before I jump into the various methods of IF and how they all work, I'm going to start by introducing a very gradual approach that is perfect for beginners and mature women. I highly recommend starting with this gradual approach so that you don't set yourself up for failure. Diving straight into an extended fast is a sure-fire way to overwhelm yourself, so start by following the below tips to ensure a smooth transition.

Start Steady and Slow

When you begin with intermittent fasting, don't jump straight into a method that involves lengthy fasts every day. Start simple; such as an overnight fast or fasting every second or third day. Once you are able to complete each fast successfully, (no cheating) then you can progress to more frequent fasts. One way of doing this is by starting off with two fasting days per week and gradually increasing the number of days by one as each week goes by. Certain diets require lengthy fasting periods of up to 36 hours, so make sure you pick a method with 14-16 hours of fasting to begin with, such as overnight fasting or the 16:8 method ("Tips for Transitioning Into Intermittent Fasting," 2020).

If you are nervous to begin fasting, you can start by slowly lengthening your time between meals. If you usually wait two to three hours between meals, try and extend this by 20-30 minutes each day; until you finally reach your goal. Ideally, you should be aiming for 5-6 hours between meals to be ready for your fasting journey. The best way to make sure that you are able to withstand long periods without food is by filling your plate with wholesome food including complex carbs, healthy fats, plenty of protein, and fruits and vegetables ("Getting Started With Intermittent Fasting," 2021).

Don't Do Too Much at Once

If you're going to start with IF, don't over-complicate things by combining it with another type of intense diet such as the ketogenic or Paleo diet (at least not in the beginning). This can really wreak havoc on your body and overwhelm it if you introduce too many changes too fast. If you're already on a keto or calorie-restricted diet, keep at it for at least two weeks before you throw IF into the mix. By introducing one new change at a time, you're making sure that your transition is not only smooth but sustainable too ("Tips for Transitioning Into Intermittent Fasting," 2020).

Pick the Right Day

If you're planning on beginning fasting for the first time, it's important that you choose an appropriate day to fast. In my experience, fasting at work is much easier than fasting at home because you're keeping your mind busy and away from thoughts of food. The worst day to begin a fast would be a weekend or a day off, as the temptation will likely be too much to withstand.

Be Sure to Eat Enough During Your Eating Window

One point that I must reiterate is to make sure that you are eating enough calories during your eating window. IF is not an excuse to simply skip meals for the purpose of cutting calories. If you severely cut your calories, you'll only slow your metabolism down and put yourself at risk for a binge after your fast is complete. Make sure that you are sticking to a healthy calorie count of at least 1200-1500 calories per day composed mainly of whole foods.

I can promise you right now that the older you get the more important your meal timing becomes, and this is especially true for those who do not incorporate any exercise into their routine. If you decide that you really need to skip a fast (for example, let's say that you typically skip breakfast), then you need to keep it high-protein and high-fat with little to no carbs. This is because you want to avoid providing your body with excess stores of glucose, as it will utilize this instead of ketones throughout the day ("Getting Started with Intermittent Fasting," 2021).

Break Your Fast Properly

Did you know that the most important meal is the one you eat to break your fast? Regardless of what time of the day your fast ends, you need to make it count. This meal should be jam-packed with protein, leafy greens, and omega-3 fats to keep your hunger hormones in check and prevent cravings throughout the day. One mistake that many people make when they start fasting is breaking their fast with too many of the wrong types of carbohydrates. This wreaks havoc on your leptin and ghrelin levels and will leave you feeling very hungry later on in the day ("Getting Started with Intermittent Fasting," 2021). If you're wondering what I mean by this, your main culprits are pastries, cookies, biscuits, white bread, and pasta. As tasty as these foods can be, they're certainly not doing your waist any favors—or your cravings!

Try Some Medium-Chain Triglyceride (MCT) Oil or Collagen Protein in the Mornings

This is one of the sneakiest and most effective tricks you can use to extend your fast for longer. Try purchasing some MCT oil or protein collagen powder to keep yourself feeling satiated throughout the day. Simply follow the serving directions on the back of the package and add a scoop to your coffee or tea when you wake up; this will keep your body in a state of ketosis for as long as possible. Protein collagen powder is especially effective at keeping your metabolism going, keeping you energized, and balancing your hormones to prevent cravings and weight gain ("Getting Started with Intermittent Fasting," 2021).

Be sure to check with a qualified healthcare consultant on the best brands of protein powder and MCT oil so that you don't waste your money. It's often better to spend a little bit more and get quality products that work rather than products that are cheap and ineffective.

Drink Plenty of Water

When you first begin your fast you'll want to make sure that you're drinking plenty of water. Not only does water help keep you full, but it will prevent you from becoming dehydrated. Some beginners to fasting experience dehydration symptoms early in their fast, as they are not receiving the fluids they normally would from certain foods. This is a major rookie error as it will throw you off your fast and trick you into thinking you're starving when you're just thirsty. Drink your H2O!

Skip Breakfast to Start

One of the easiest tried and tested methods for beginners is simply skipping breakfast, eating your first meal at noon, and filling up on tea and coffee. Trust me, it's a lot easier than you think! If your goal is weight loss then all you need to do is eat a healthy, low-carb lunch and dinner and try to eat your last meal before 7:00 p.m. Here is what an ideal fasting schedule would look like for beginners:

- Eat your last meal around 7:00 p.m. (8:00 p.m. at the absolute latest).

- Fast until noon (you can fill up on black coffee and tea).

- Break your fast by enjoying a low-carb lunch with plenty of leafy greens, protein, and a small number of complex carbs (quinoa, brown rice, etc).

- Eat a wholesome, healthy dinner around 6:00-7:00 p.m., and repeat the process until noon the following day.

The great thing about this method is that you spend half of your fast sleeping, meaning the other half will fly by much faster; however, this is only one way of doing it. There are plenty of other safe and effective methods that you can use, which brings me to the next chapter.

CHAPTER 4

EIGHT OF THE MOST EFFECTIVE METHODS OF FASTING: EXPLAINED!

Now that you're clued up on everything to do with fasting, it's time to get started on the most important part—choosing your method! In this chapter, I've outlined eight of the most effective methods with a list of pros and cons to make the decision easier for you. Remember to choose a method that best suits your lifestyle by comparing your daily schedule with how your fast would fit in. With all this in mind, let's get started!

A Precautionary Word

Before I dive into this, it's important to mention that women may react differently to fasting than men do so we need to be extra careful. Our bodies are far more sensitive to signals of starvation as we are naturally designed for childbirth. Because of this, our hormones can very easily be thrown out of kilter when fasting is involved—according to what experts have to say on the matter. This information is based on one specific study conducted on rats, whereby the female rats experienced adverse effects on their fertility when fasting.

But, as other experts say, the anatomy and metabolism of a rat is vastly different from that of a human. It would be inaccurate to say that the findings from one isolated study on rats can be used as proof that fasting affects women differently to men, so we can only speculate. If you are still concerned, then it's best to start with a method specifically designed for women and work your way up from there.

The Crescendo Method

This involves shorter fasts of 12-16 hours maximum. Funnily enough, you've probably done this a few times without even being aware which proves how simple it is! Not only are the fasting hours shorter, but you're only required to fast two to three days per week non-consecutively (Taylor, 2017). For example, you can choose to fast Monday, Wednesday, and Friday and start your fast at 8:00 p.m., eating again around 9:00-10:00 a.m. the following morning. That's very doable!

Pros vs Cons

As the name suggests, you'll gradually increase the number of hours that you choose to fast as your body slowly adapts. Since women tend to have a harder time adapting to changes in the body, this is a great option to ease into things. You definitely don't want to add any unnecessary stress to your body, so crescendo fasting could be a great option that won't wreak havoc on your hunger hormones. You'll still be following the fasting lifestyle and you'll still lose weight, but you're not going to the extreme. This allows for a much smoother transition into your fasting regime, which will inevitably boost your confidence and self-belief.

In terms of the cons, there's very few negatives to this method. If you find that your weight loss is too slow you can always increase the frequency of days spent fasting or the hours. You can think of this as a baseline to start, and slowly work your way up from there.

The Leangains or 16/8 Method

This second method is one of the most common and was popularized by Martin Berkhan, a well-known nutritionist, author, and personal trainer. If you are someone who is relatively active and hits the Zumba classes, then this could be an ideal method for you. Even if you aren't an avid gym-goer, this method is ideal for women wanting to lose fat and gain muscle (which should be the ultimate goal)! Essentially, you can follow this method by fasting for 14-16 hours and then eat all your calories within an eight-hour window. That said, experts recommend that women benefit more from 14-hour fasts, so I would consider opting for this length of time.

The easiest way to follow this method is by eating your last meal in the evenings, sleeping through most of the fast, and eating your next meal around noon. You can play around with the times of your last meal and the next, as long as you complete your 14-hour fast. For example, you could eat your last meal at 8:00 p.m. and then eat the following day at 10:00 p.m. to have successfully completed the leangains fast. Bet you didn't think it was so easy? Well, there's a little more to it when you incorporate exercise—which is incredibly important.

On the days that you choose to work out, make sure that you are eating a sufficient amount of carbohydrates to provide you with the fuel your body needs to execute a workout properly. The best carbs to eat on your non-rest days are brown rice, whole wheat bread, quinoa, whole grains, beans, and vegetables. As women over 50, it's unlikely that you're going to be benching 100-pound weights, but it's still important to fuel your body for a brisk walk or swim. On your resting days, you should prioritize your protein and fat intake while minimizing carbs as much as possible. This is because your body doesn't need the extra glucose when you aren't significantly active, so it will end up being stored as fat. The protein and fat will keep your body in ketosis and feed your muscles while they rest so you don't lose precious muscle mass.

Pros vs Cons

One of the biggest advantages of this method is its simplicity. The eight-hour eating window is relatively long compared to other methods, meaning you have more freedom to eat when you please. This makes it great for social ladies or women who want to plan their weeks and easily fit fasting into the equation.

In terms of the cons, you really need to eat healthy, wholesome foods or this method won't work. You also need to make sure that you do not accidentally break your fast by adding sugar or whole milk to your coffee and tea! While it's perfectly okay to enjoy some black coffee, tea, or water during your fast, make sure that you leave out any unexpected calories.

The 5/2 Method

This option was first made popular in 2013 by a well-known British journalist called Michael Mosley and is also known as the "Fast Diet." As the name suggests, this diet involves eating normally five days of the week and fasting for the remaining two. Sounds pretty straightforward, right? Well, the caveat is that you can only eat 500-600 calories on your fasting days, which is pretty limited. For women, Mosley suggests only 500 calories while men should allow 600. The good news is that you don't need to fast for two days consecutively, you can split your fasting days evenly throughout the week so that you don't feel hungry or weak (Gunnars, 2021).

For example, you may choose to fast on Tuesdays and Thursdays and eat normally for the rest of the week. You can split your meals up as you wish—for example, you could split your calories into three 200 calorie meals or two 300 calorie meals on your fasting days (Gunnars, 2021). It's entirely up to you!

Pros vs Cons

The great thing about this method is the fact that you have the freedom to eat as you please for five days of the week. When I say this, I don't mean going crazy with cakes and chocolates; you should be eating three healthy meals per day. This method of fasting boosts a large range of health benefits, such as decreased blood pressure, improved cognitive functioning, cholesterol, and insulin. It also allows you to have a relatively open social schedule, as you only need to set aside two days of restrictions rather than every day.

In terms of the cons, you're probably already thinking of one! Eating only 500-600 calories per day is an extremely low number, and not everyone can sustain this in the long term. While some ladies may cope just fine, others may really struggle with weakness and cravings. It's up to you to decide how much your body can withstand and what you're typically accustomed to.

Eat Stop Eat

This method was first made known by well-known fitness expert Brad Pilon and appears to be quite a popular option. That said, it's certainly not for the fainthearted. Essentially, you'll be choosing one or two days per week where you fast for 24-hours straight. During this 24-hour period, you may only consume low-calorie tea, coffee, or water with absolutely no solid foods allowed. One way of doing this would be to begin your fast at 8:00 p.m. and only eat again at 8:00 p.m. the following night, meaning you've successfully completed a full 24-hour fast. Once your fast is over you can resume eating. Make sure that you break your fast with wholesome foods that contain plenty of vitamins and minerals and *do not* restrict your calories during your eating window—you should be eating the same number of calories you normally would before you fast.

If you feel as though 24-hours is too long, you can always start off with 18-hours and slowly work your way up. As a beginner, it's not a good idea to jump all-in to 24-hours, as a rule.

Pros vs Cons

The best part about this diet is the fact that you can really enjoy and savor the foods you love once your fast is over. While 24-hours is a long time to go without food, you'll be able to eat all the foods you love once the fast is complete to compensate. While you shouldn't go crazy and eat an entire tub of ice cream, you can happily enjoy some pizza, chocolate, and other carbohydrates in moderation. You won't need to obsess over counting calories nor will you have any forbidden foods, making this a massive perk! Plus, you're more likely to reach the autophagy stage using this method than you would with the others.

In terms of the cons, 24-hours is an extremely long time to go without food. As a result, there's a higher chance of you experiencing unpleasant symptoms such as headaches, fatigue, and grumpiness. Lastly, you may feel so hungry after your fast that you end up binging afterward, which isn't healthy either.

The Warrior Diet

This next method was started by Ori Hofmeklr, one of the pioneers of intermittent fasting. He graduated with a degree in Human Sciences, and served in the military, which inspired him to learn more about the mechanisms of survival and how stress affects the body. While this method isn't the That said, this diet could be ideal for someone who doesn't eat much during the day and consumes the majority of their calories in the evenings. Essentially, The Warrior Diet involves fasting for 20 hours per day with a small eating window of only four hours. The idea behind this method is that we are all nocturnal beings and need to remain in sync with our circadian rhythms in order to stay slim, alert, and allow fat burning to be boosted. With this method you are permitted to snack on fruits and vegetables during your fast, but nothing substantial.

Your four-hour eating window should take place in the evenings where you eat one large meal composed mainly of whole, unprocessed foods. Hofmeklr recommends eating in the evenings as he believes this improves hormone regulation and fat burning during the day. He also believes that the order in which you eat your food groups makes a difference, recommending that you start with vegetables, followed by protein, and then fat. If you are still hungry after this, only then can you move on to carbohydrates.

Pros vs Cons

Compared to Eat Stop Eat, this method has its advantages because you can snack throughout the day; this makes a huge difference in energy levels and sustainability. This method also boasts some really impressive results in terms of energy levels and fat loss, which is a major advantage.

In terms of the cons, this method may be difficult for those who don't enjoy eating one huge meal in the evenings. For example, if you suffer from indigestion or heartburn, this method is probably not going to work for you. You also need to be aware of the foods that you snack on, as you could end up gaining weight if you eat too much of the wrong thing during the day. This means you would need to be more stringent with the foods you eat in comparison to other methods.

Alternate-Day Fasting

Alternate-day fasting is on the extreme side of the fasting spectrum, but its benefits appear to make up for the extremity! This method was first popularized by James Johnson, M.D., and involves alternating between feasting and fasting. Researchers have been paying particular attention to alternate-day fasting due to its popularity, with the intent to find out exactly how beneficial this diet really is. Alternate-day fasting is also known as the "Every Other Day Diet" which has been widely studied and published by Professor Krista Varady, a fasting enthusiast. As the name suggests, this diet involves fasting for one day and then eating normally the next, continuing this pattern throughout the week. On your fasting days you don't need to refrain from food all together, but rather limit your calorie intake to the specified requirements as mentioned earlier (Mann, 2021).

For example, this is what your week could look like:

- Monday (normal eating)
- Tuesday (fasting with a limit of 500 calories)
- Wednesday (normal eating)
- Thursday (fasting with a limit of 500 calories)
- Friday (normal eating)
- Saturday (fasting with a limit of 500 calories)
- Sunday (normal eating)

The calories that you consume on your fasting days should contain approximately 50 grams of protein to preserve energy, muscle, and keep you feeling fuller for longer. You can also enjoy low-calorie beverages. On your non-fasting days, you're free to enjoy any type of food as long as you keep an eye on your calorie count. According to Varady, this isn't something you need to worry about, as studies have shown that people following this diet only consume 10% more calories on their non-fasting days (Mann, 2021).

Pros vs Cons

In terms of efficacy, people following this method appear to lose between 10 and 15 pounds within three months. When compared to other types of fasting that involve daily eating windows, these results are far superior. Studies conducted by Professor Varady have shown that this method of fasting is more likely to induce autophagy than other methods, and also helps to prevent type 2 diabetes. In the studies, followers of this diet experienced lowered insulin and blood pressure which both contribute to the development of diabetes when left unchecked (Mann, 2021).

Additional studies have found that cutting your calories down by 20%-35% of your usual intake can result in a weight loss of two and a half pounds per week (Morin, 2017). That's impressive!

As with everything in life, there are always drawbacks. Studies on this form of fasting show that it has the highest dropout rate of all the other methods, and it's not hard to see why (Mann, 2021). Calorie-counting every second day can be tedious, and it's hard to plan your life around this when you're needing to fast every second day of the week. It's very easy to delay a fast due to temptation, end up messing up your schedule for the week and need to start again. You really need to have the willpower to succeed at this method.

Spontaneous Meal Skipping

This method is by far the easiest one to follow due to its sheer simplicity. If you are feeling uncertain about IF and are looking to ease your way into it then this is definitely the method for you. In order to follow this method you simply need to listen to your body's hunger and fullness cues, which involves a mindful approach. For example, have you ever eaten a meal simply for the sake of it? As humans, we are habitual creatures and we have programmed our bodies to eat at certain times of the day even if we aren't necessarily hungry. With spontaneous meal skipping you will simply skip a meal every so often when you don't feel genuinely hungry.

Over time you will develop a calorie deficit which will eventually lead to weight loss—without much effort. Instead of forcing breakfast down when you're late for work or eating dinner simply because everyone else is, skip that meal and reap the incredible benefits. That said, you should not make a habit of skipping meals every single day. Studies have shown that when you skip meals every now and again in conjunction with a healthy diet, you're more likely to lose weight and remain healthy (Parker-Pope, 2007).

Pros vs Cons

Skipping meals (breakfast in particular) certainly has more benefits than drawbacks. Skipping breakfast can help to control blood sugar, reduce fat, insulin resistance, and bad cholesterol. Human trials conducted by the University of Surrey examined two groups of healthy individuals all eating the same healthy foods. They wanted to discover whether the timing of the meals made any difference, and they discovered that those who skipped breakfast—or waited for an extra 90 minutes before digging in—had lower body fat, blood sugar, and cholesterol than the other group ("The Pros and Cons of Skipping Breakfast," 2021).

In terms of the drawbacks, I'm pretty hard-pressed to find anything. That said, if you do have a pre-existing condition such as diabetes or you are pregnant, then meal skipping isn't a good option; additionally, meal skipping may not be feasible for people who are very active on a daily basis and need constant fuel. Besides that, meal skipping is generally an easy, viable option for most people.

Overnight Fasting or 12-Hour Fasting

Lastly, overnight fasting is another incredibly simple and effective method. All you need to do is refrain from late-night snacking and finish your last meal as early in the evening as possible. According to the University of California's school of medicine, overnight fasting can help to reduce the risk of developing breast cancer. Since this method of fasting helps to control blood sugar over a long period of time, the risk of cancer is automatically decreased. On top of this, overnight or 12-hour fasting is much better for women's hormones and metabolism (Entin, 2015).

Overnight fasts provide your body with the opportunity to burn through sugar stores, otherwise known as glycogen. When you're indulging in midnight snacks, you're not giving your body the chance to eat through your fat stores and regulate other important bodily functions. Fasting during the night also helps your body eliminate excess salt which can contribute to hypertension ("What Is Intermittent Fasting and Does it Really Work," 2021).

The great thing about this method is the fact that you're splitting your eating and fasting windows up evenly and you spend the vast majority of your fasting window sleeping. In order to successfully complete a 12-hour fast, you'll need to make sure that you finish your last meal before the 12-hour fasting and non-fasting intervals. For example, if you are planning to fast from 7:00 p.m. to 7:00 a.m., then you must make sure that you eat breakfast just after seven in the morning and eat your last meal before seven in the evening (Tabahlia, 2021).

Pros vs Cons

12-hour fasts are a safer option for older women who are new to fasting as they won't cause a dramatic change in blood sugar or hormones. They are also much easier to follow and stick to and can be used as a gateway method to the more challenging types of intermittent fasting.

In terms of the cons, you may not see results as quickly as you would with more extreme methods of fasting. If you're looking for a more dramatic change in your weight, then this method may be too slow for you. You'll also need to make sure that you carefully monitor the calories that you eat; otherwise, you will override the benefits of the overnight fast.

The Bottom Line

If you're feeling a little overwhelmed by all the different options, that's completely normal; each method has its own set of benefits and drawbacks that you need to weigh up for yourself to make an informed decision. Once you've reached your decision, it's time to move onto the most exciting part—getting started! The great thing about IF is that you don't need to stick to one method. If you feel that one isn't working for you, you can always choose a different method and see how that goes until you find the perfect fit.

CHAPTER 5

EIGHT EFFECTIVE METHODS OF FASTING: GETTING STARTED WITH A COMPREHENSIVE GUIDE

Now that you're aware of the various types of fasting, it's time to dive deeper into how you can implement your method of choice into your lifestyle. In this chapter, you'll find a step-by-step comprehensive guide explaining how each method works so that you know exactly what to do throughout your journey. With all this in mind, let's get started!

Special Note for Women

While I have mentioned this earlier, I must reiterate that women may react differently to fasting than men do. This means that we need to take extra special care in listening to our bodies and treating them with respect and understanding. Women who practice longer fasts tend to experience worsened blood sugar and insulin levels when compared to men, so shorter fasts are safer and more effective. Always start off with the simplest of methods and slowly ease your way into this new pattern of eating.

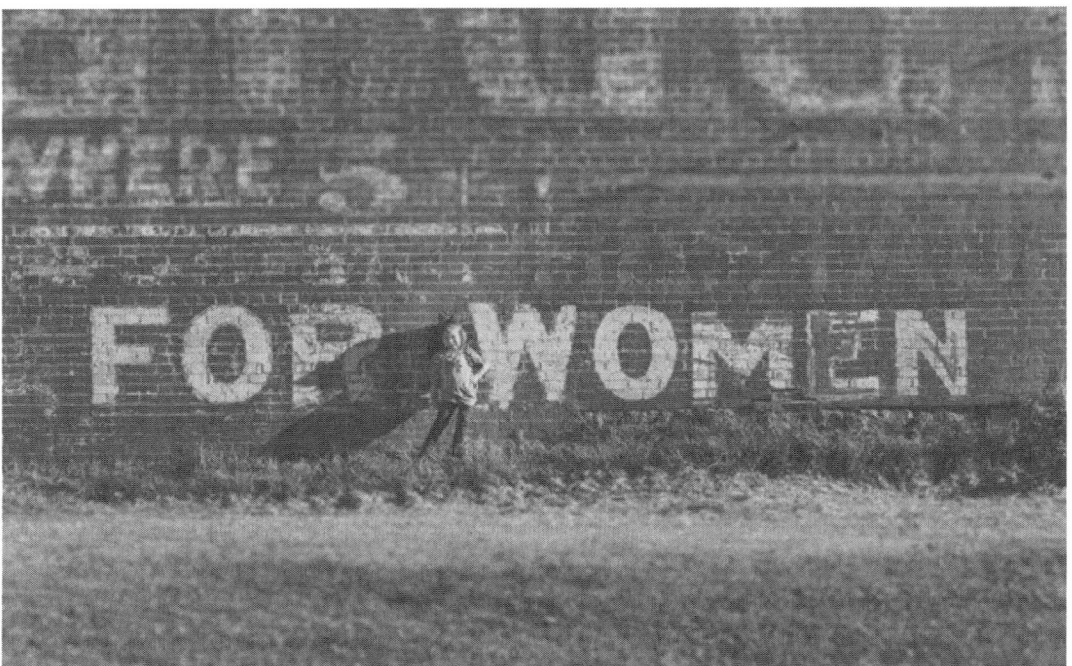

If you experience discomfort aside from the initial hunger pangs, you should stop or see a doctor.

With all this in mind, most concerns tend to come from younger women. This is because younger people need to consume more calories than their elders for several reasons, so they feel the repercussions of fasting more than someone older than them. As an example, my 62-year old mom only eats once per day, and she's never heard of intermittent fasting in her life! As we grow older we need fewer calories to sustain us; especially when we aren't moving around as much as we used to. This is why IF can be a really convenient and successful method for older women, as it seems to make more sense and fit in better with their lifestyles.

The Crescendo Method

Choosing Your Days

You've decided on the Crescendo method of fasting—good choice! Now that you know the basics of how this method works it's time to dive into the nitty-gritty of things. As a beginner, it's a wise choice to start with a two-day plan and work your way up from there. So, you'll need to decide which two days will suit you best by looking at your schedule. For example, do you usually go for breakfast on Sundays or do you and your family have a late-night snacking tradition on Saturdays? These are the days that you should opt out for your fasting days, as you know the chances of breaking the fast are significantly higher.

Choose days that you know will have the fewest temptations such as a busy Tuesday morning where you'll likely skip breakfast anyway. Plus, you'll have fewer temptations on a Monday night than a Sunday night—we all know how it goes. Any day from Monday to Thursday should be your easiest day to fast, but you can choose whichever day you feel most comfortable with.

Choosing Your Hours

Next, you need to choose how many hours you're comfortable fasting for. If you're a beginner and you're nervous about making a mistake, then start with a simple 12-hour fast for the first week. This means that you could start your fast at 8:00 p.m. and have your first cup of coffee and snack the following morning at 8:00 a.m. This is really easy to do and you shouldn't find yourself struggling too hard to stick to this plan; you just need to make sure that you stick to water only after 8:00 p.m., as anything with calories will break your fast. When you wake up, be sure to drink a glass of warm water with lemon to get your digestion going. You may even find that drinking sufficient water in the morning allows you to extend your fast for longer than 12-hours, so give that a try!

Choosing Your Food

In order to refrain from that after-dinner snack that you'll likely be craving, you'll need to make sure that your dinner was sufficient. A well-balanced meal of fiber, protein, complex carbs, and healthy fats is your best option. All these combined will help to keep you full and your calories in check.

For example, an excellent dinner option would be lean pesto chicken, brown rice, broccoli, and beans. You're getting a full dose of complex carbs to keep you satiated, plenty of protein, and healthy fats from the pesto. Because this is such a well-rounded, nutrient-dense meal, you're far less likely to break your fast and indulge in midnight-snacking.

Exercise

Trust me, I get it. As we grow older, exercise is the *last* thing on our minds and the mere thought of putting on track pants and going for a run sounds like a torture; nevertheless, exercise makes you look and feel incredible, plus you'll reach your weight loss goals a whole lot quicker. The great thing about this particular method is the fact that you are able to exercise as much as you please due to the shorter fasting periods and timing of the fasts.

For older women, some lightweight training and cardio are perfect for maintaining cardiovascular health, preventing muscle loss, and keeping fit and healthy. If you can, schedule your workouts on your non-fasting days, especially if you are doing a 16-hour fast. That said, a simple 12-hour fast shouldn't affect your ability to exercise whatsoever. Ideally, you can do some light cardio such as swimming and jogging on your fasting days and engage in weight training on your non-fasting days. It's always a good idea to incorporate some form of exercise into your daily routine to get your blood pumping, energy levels boosted, and endorphins flowing! Remember, a 20-minute light walk is better than nothing at all.

Hydration

While I've mentioned this before, I cannot stress the importance of keeping hydrated. Try and aim for 10-12 glasses of water every day; avoid fizzy drinks and alcohol if you can (trust me, they're not doing your waistline *any* favors). Alcoholic and carbonated drinks will also dehydrate you much quicker, so make sure that you consume an extra glass of water for every alcoholic or carbonated beverage you consume.

The Leangains or 16/8 Method

This next method is one of my personal favorites for women as it's easy to follow and super effective. The 16/8 method is very similar to the crescendo method except the recommended fasting hours are slightly longer with this one; the aim is to practice fasting every day. If this seems a little overwhelming, you can always start with the crescendo method and gradually work your way to the 16/8 technique once you feel more comfortable and your body has adapted.

Choosing Your Days

For this method you'll be fasting every day of the week, Monday through Sunday (or at least this is what you will strive for). It's perfectly okay to miss a fasting day here and there, especially if you have a special occasion coming up. That said, try not to make a habit of this as consistency is vital for your fasting journey's success! I always like to say that missing a day of exercise, eating badly, or staying in bed is human, and it won't do any harm to our goals or livelihoods. But, when you do this for two days in a row you're creating an unhealthy pattern. So, what's the takeaway? Essentially, you're allowed one day of slacking but no more; otherwise, you're setting a negative mindset and pattern of behavior.

Choosing Your Hours

As the name suggests, the 16/8 method involves fasting for 16 hours of the day and eating for the remaining 8. For women, experts recommend that women follow a 14-hour fast, as this is safer and more effective (but you can choose what feels best for you). When it comes to your hours, most people decide to fast in the morning and resume their eating window from lunchtime through dinner. There are a few reasons for this, but typically people are busier in the mornings and more relaxed in the later afternoon, meaning that they prefer to eat most of their daily calories during this time. Personally, I find it much easier to fast in the mornings, and my energy levels are boosted when I haven't eaten a big breakfast; however, everyone is different and there are alternative ways of following the 16/8 method.

For example, you may set your eating window between 10:00 a.m. and 6:00 p.m. (a full eight hours). This is another great way of fasting as you can enjoy a decent breakfast, a light lunch, and snacks, as well as an early dinner while still sticking to the recommended eating window. You're getting in all three meals within this time and you're spending the majority of your fast sleeping, which is definitely a bonus! That said, the most common way to follow the 16/8 method is by setting your eating window from noon until 8:00 p.m. and then fasting all the way through to noon again the following day (Link, 2018).

If you're not sure how to begin, the best thing to do is analyze your typical eating patterns. Do you usually eat a lot in the evenings but don't enjoy heavy meals in the morning? Then you should set your eating window from noon until later in the evening. Conversely, if you often find yourself starving in the mornings but suffer from heartburn after a heavy evening meal, then you'll naturally choose the alternative option. The great thing about the 16/8 method is that you can switch around the times to suit your lifestyle, as long as you make sure you have an eating window of 8 hours and you fast for the remaining 14-16. It's as simple as that!

Choosing Your Food

When it comes to your dietary choices, the 16/8 method requires a healthy, balanced diet of whole grains, protein, healthy fats, fruits, and of course, vegetables. In terms of your whole grains, you should be eating brown rice, buckwheat, barley, oats, quinoa, and whole-grain pasta. White bread, cookies, cakes, and other artificial carbs are a big no-no! In terms of protein, you should be eating a combination of eggs, chicken, fish, legumes, nuts, seeds, and a moderate dose of red meat. I know that most people think that red meat is 'bad,' but everything is fine in moderation (Link, 2018). That said, you shouldn't be eating it every day, but once or twice a week is perfectly okay!

As part of a healthy, balanced diet you should also be eating plenty of fresh fruits and vegetables. Not only are they fiber-rich and low-calorie, but many of them contain disease-fighting and anti-aging antioxidants. Foods with the most antioxidants are blueberries, broccoli (great for your fiber intake), potatoes, avocadoes, carrots, collard greens, kale, cabbage, and chia seeds (to name a few). Apples, pears, oranges, strawberries, and bananas are also excellent snacks to fill the gap between meals (Link, 2018). If you're really looking for the best low-calorie snack, strawberries contain as few as four calories per berry, which is virtually nothing! Plus, they're juicy, succulent, and delicious.

When it comes to fat, many women panic and immediately assume that it should be avoided at all costs. Truthfully, fats are a vital part of your diet and you should be incorporating them as part of your daily meal plan. What really matters is which types of fats you are eating, as there are different varieties that can be categorized as either 'good' or 'bad' fats. There are four main types of fats, namely: saturated, polyunsaturated, trans fats, and monounsaturated fats. Saturated and trans fats are considered unhealthy and should be consumed in small portions, so you should always check the labels on your food and make sure that these levels of fat are low.

Some common examples of these two types of bad fats are: greasy fried foods, margarine, microwave popcorn, baked goods, and vegetable shortening—which is commonly used to cook and bake with. If you've never heard of vegetable shortening, it's simply a cheap substitute for butter and is a partially hydrogenated form of vegetable oil. It's commonly used due to its incredibly high-fat content that allows for a much softer pastry when compared to alternatives such as butter (Coyle, 2017).

Healthy fats that you should be eating are avocados, coconut oil, and olive oil. Your body needs these fats to keep your body functioning optimally and keep your energy levels up. Healthy fats are also packed with vitamins and minerals. That said, replace the unhealthy oils in your pantry with coconut and olive oil, and use these when you cook instead. Don't be shy to slice up some avocado and have it with your breakfast or lunch on the side. While they may be a higher-calorie fruit, you're getting all the good fats and antioxidants and you'll feel fuller for much longer, meaning you'll eat less throughout the day.

Exercise

When it comes to the 16/8 method, the best time to get some exercise is first thing in the morning while you are still in a fasted state. Since most people choose to fast from dinner to noon the next day, you can hit a walk, swim, or jog as soon as you wake up. The reason behind this is due to our natural circadian rhythms—it's always better to exercise in the morning than the evening, as this can disrupt the quality of your sleep, particularly the REM stage (Rapid Eye Movement) which is crucial for many vital brain activities.

Some people are nervous to exercise on an empty stomach as they believe that this is damaging to the metabolism and causes muscle loss, but this simply isn't true. Exercising in a fasted state helps to maximize the benefits of exercise and fasting in what is known as a multi-therapeutic approach ("Working Out While Intermittent Fasting," 2021). Plus, you won't experience uncomfortable cramps!

Studies have shown that waiting two to three hours before you eat after a workout results in a rise in HGH (Human Growth Hormone) which promotes fat burning and encourages the body to use stored glucose as energy. This is all because the body has developed adaptive mechanisms to handle hunger post-workout, and this is exactly how your body copes. Most importantly, you will want to avoid heavy workouts when waiting two to three hours before eating. Light walks, jogging, and some lightweight lifting are the perfect options. If you do decide to do heavy cardio, then you should prepare an immediate post-workout meal to avoid feeling dizzy, lightheaded, or weak ("Working Out While Intermittent Fasting," 2021).

Hydration

As with any diet, keeping yourself hydrated is absolutely key. With the 16/8 method, you are free to enjoy black coffee, tea, or any other zero-calorie beverage during your fast. Personally, coffee and tea are my go-to drinks during my morning fast to keep my stomach full and my mind stimulated! Green tea is an excellent morning drink to get your energy levels up without the coffee jitters, and some people find that green tea is a natural appetite suppressant.

The 5:2 Method

The 5:2 method is significantly different from the first two methods in that you're eating normally most of the time with only two days spent fasting—that's the good part! The tough part is the calorie restriction on your fasting days. To be more accurate, proponents of this diet say that you should aim to eat 25% of your normal daily calories on your fasting days. So, if you normally eat 2000 calories, then 25% of that would be 500. If you normally eat fewer than that, then you would adjust this accordingly. That said, there's no need to worry as I'm going to outline how you can easily follow this method without feeling too hungry or deprived. Let's get started!

Choosing Your Days

When it comes to your fasting and non-fasting days, you'll want to choose wisely. If you get this part wrong, then the rest will fall apart! Essentially, you'll want to choose your busiest days for fasting. For example, a bad fasting day to choose would be a lazy Saturday or Sunday where you know you'll want to snack, or perhaps you have a lavish dinner planned. You're setting yourself up for failure if you choose days that you know will present more temptation than necessary.

That said, some good fasting days are Monday to Thursday, as most people are busy working and have enough distractions to turn their minds away from the thought of mindlessly eating. Personally, I naturally fast on workdays as I don't have time to make breakfast in the mornings, and I fill up on coffee at work when I'm busy. The fast happens naturally!

Secondly, you will want to split these days up with at least one day in between your fasting days. Trust me, fasting two days consecutively is *not* the best way to get through this! For example, you could choose Monday and Thursday as your fasting days. This gives you two days in between for normal eating, meaning you'll have plenty of time to prepare and fuel up for your next fast.

Choosing Your Hours

In terms of your hours, you can eat whenever you like on both your fasting and non-fasting days. The key is to make sure that you stick to your calorie limit on your fasting days—how you choose to ensure this is done is entirely up to you. Personally, I find that eating breakfast early in the morning causes me to feel hungrier throughout the day; therefore, making me eat more calories. For others, breakfast may be the key meal to provide energy to get through the day without feeling too hungry. Depending on which category you fall into, you can decide whether or not you'll have breakfast on your fasting days.

According to Marengo (2019), you could set your eating plan out in the following ways:

- Eating one large meal in the evening
- Eating a small breakfast, lunch, and light dinner
- Eating a small breakfast, late lunch, and skipping dinner
- Eating an early lunch and early dinner

You can play around with these and see which method works best for you. If you do choose to eat three meals per day, bear in mind that these meals will have to be extremely small. That said, it may be easier to cut your meals down to at least two on your fasting days so that you can eat a more substantial portion in one sitting.

Choosing Your Food

Since you're eating such a small quantity on fasting days, you'll need to select your meals very wisely. Ultimately, your food choices should be rich in fiber and nutrients with filling properties. In terms of energy and satiety, protein is your best friend! While you can enjoy fattier meats on your non-fasting days, you'll want to stick to lean protein on your fasting days. Examples of lean protein options are: white fish, beans, poultry, peas, eggs, lentils, tofu, and any other lean animal cut. When preparing these options, try and avoid frying them as this adds extra calories and fat. Baking, grilling, boiling, or roasting are your healthier options, so bear that in mind when you're cooking (Marengo, 2019).

Leafy greens and fruits are also excellent, as you can pile your plate with them and still enjoy a low-calorie count. It's better to have a huge plate of healthy food over a tiny plate of higher-calorie foods, so try and plan your meals with this in mind. One easy way of filling your plate (and your tummy) is by investing in a spiralizer. You can use this to transform zucchini, cauliflower, and carrots into a type of pasta that you can enjoy guilt-free and it's much tastier than you think (Marengo, 2019).

Soup is another excellent option for your fasting days as it's packed with nutrition and generally very low in calories. Since it's liquid, you'll also feel fuller after a bowl of soup—another bonus! Chicken, vegetable, butternut, and lentil soup are all excellent examples of healthy soups you can prepare from scratch or purchase from the store. If you're wondering what your meal plan for a fasting day could look like, here's a prime example:

- Two hard boiled eggs for breakfast (160 calories).

- One serving of vegetable soup for lunch.
- Steamed white fish medallion with a large portion of steamed vegetables for dinner (300 calories).

On your regular days, it is important not to binge or use these as cheat days. While you can eat more calories than on your non-fasting days, they should be composed of wholesome, nutrient-rich foods. Gorging on fried, greasy foods and cakes on your non-fasting days will render your two-day fast futile, so don't do it! So, if you usually eat 1,500 calories per day, make sure that this is made up of protein, healthy fats, complex carbs, and plenty of fruits and vegetables (Marengo, 2019). Remember, this isn't only about weight loss—eating like this is beneficial for your overall health and wellbeing in promoting a longer, happier life.

Hydration

Similar to the other methods, you should stick to zero-calorie beverages such as tea, coffee, and water. One thing I must mention is that you should not drink zero-calorie energy drinks such as sugar-free Redbull and Coke Zero. This is because these drinks are packed with aspartame and other synthetic ingredients that mimic the taste of sugar, which can break your fast despite the fact that they don't contain any calories. Why? Well, these drinks trick your body into thinking that you're consuming sugar, so your insulin and blood sugar levels respond accordingly, affecting your fasted state. I made this mistake myself when fasting, and only found out later down the line that I was unknowingly breaking my fast! Don't make the same mistake.

Eat Stop Eat

Similar to the 5:2 method, this next one involves eating normally for five to six days of the week and then fasting for one or two non-consecutive days. What differentiates this method from the above is the severity of the fast—for this method, you'll be going without food for a *full* 24 hours. If you think you've got what it takes, this method can be a highly effective way to shed visceral fat and reap the full benefits of intermittent fasting. The best part about this diet is that it's straightforward and does not involve much planning, just simple execution. Let's dive in!

Choosing Your Days

Logically, you'll want to arrange your 24-hour fast on a day where you'll have the least temptations. Not only that, but you also need the right balance of busy and relaxed. Abstaining from food for an entire day is not an easy feat, especially if you are new to the fasting game. For example, if you know that you usually have big meetings on Fridays or you generally go for a walk or jog on Sundays, then you'll want to eliminate the idea of fasting for 24-hours on those days. Whether you fast for one or two days per week is entirely up to you—if you are a beginner, it's best to start with one day per week and work your way up from there.

You just need to make sure that you are not unknowingly fasting for longer than 24-hours. For example, if you begin your fast at 10:00 a.m. on Wednesday and plan to end it at the same time on Thursday, you need to make sure that you eat a good meal just before 10:00 a.m. on Wednesday. This will not only help carry you through your fast, but ensure you're not fasting for too long (Coyle, 2020).

Choosing Your Hours

For this particular method, the answer is pretty straightforward—you'll be fasting for 24 hours! The only thing you need to decide is your start and end time, and this is entirely up to you. For example, you may decide that you would like to begin your fast at noon and end it at noon the following day. This will give you enough time to eat two meals before the beginning of your fast to help sustain you through to your next eating window. If you choose to begin your fast earlier, you have the benefit of breaking it earlier the next day but you have less time to fuel up in preparation.

Choosing Your Food

When it comes to the eat stop eat diet, you're creating a substantial calorie deficit when you fast for a full 24 hours, even if it's only once per week. So, you need to make sure that when you do eat you are eating wholesome, nutrient-rich foods. Before you begin your 24-hour fast, you should eat a variety of low-GI complex carbohydrates to keep you fuller for longer and balance your blood sugar levels in preparation for your fast. According to Coyle (2020), some examples of low-GI foods include the following:

- rye and sourdough bread
- whole-grain bread
- steel-cut oats and bran
- celery, zucchini, carrots, broccoli, and cauliflower
- milk, cheese, soy milk, almond milk, and yogurt
- all types of fruits
- sweet potatoes, yams, squash, and corn
- brown and basmati rice
- the entire legume family, including chickpeas (hummus), lentils, baked beans, and kidney beans

These are some of the best examples of low-GI foods, but there are certainly more! Eating these before you begin your fast is an excellent way to ensure you have a safe, effective fast.

As a side note, if you find that you are not losing weight then it is recommended that you reduce your calorie intake on non-fasting days by 10% (Horton, 2021).

Exercise

You can exercise on the eat stop eat method, but Brad Pilon suggests low-impact cardio such as walking, jogging, and swimming. Pilon is one of the leading advocates for the benefits of intermittent fasting, and has a graduate degree in Human Biology and Nutritional Sciences. He emphasizes building muscle, fat loss, improving health, and approaching weight loss through a permanent change in lifestyle. That said, he also suggests that resistance and low-impact weight training is important for muscle building and stimulation. For older women especially, it's not a good idea to do high-impact exercises such as running while on this diet, and exercise should be avoided completely on fasting days (Horton, 2021).

Instead, practice some low-impact weight training and light cardio once you have eaten, and don't push your body too hard.

Hydration

On your fasting days, it is more important than ever that you drink plenty of water to avoid dehydration. As mentioned earlier, you are more susceptible to dehydration when you fast as you are not receiving water in the foods you would normally eat throughout the day. As a rule, coffee and tea are always permitted as they not only help to keep you stimulated but are natural appetite suppressants. Just make sure you don't add any extra sugar or creamer as this will break your fast!

The Warrior Diet

This next fasting method is for those ladies who prefer to eat very little during the day and eat larger meals in the evenings. If you have a busy lifestyle and prefer to graze, then this could be a really convenient option. Personally, I know a few women who really battle to eat large meals too late in the evenings as they suffer from heartburn and indigestion. If you fall under this category then this method may not be the one for you. Essentially, you're following a 20/4 schedule—fasting for 20 hours per day and eating for the remaining 4. Do you think you're up to the challenge? Here's what to do.

Choosing Your Days

The great thing about this method is the fact that you can eat whatever you want during your four-hour eating window. Pizza, pasta, ice cream, or french fries—the choice is yours! Another benefit is the fact that you don't have to completely abstain from all food during your 20-hour fast. You are allowed boiled eggs, dairy, fruits and vegetables, and low-calorie drinks. If this sounds a little bit overwhelming, we've outlined what a typical day on this method may look like on the following page. For now, you just need to know that this method should—ideally—be followed every day of the week.

As a side note, it's important to understand that while you are allowed to go crazy on your choice of food at night, the choices you make will influence how much weight you lose and how quickly. If you eat pizza and pasta every night, the weight loss will be significantly slower than if you ate a big, wholesome meal of protein, starch, and vegetables. That said, if you follow this diet correctly, you stand to lose between 10-15 pounds per week. Choose wisely!

Choosing Your Hours

The easiest way to do this would be to choose which time in the evening you would prefer to open your eating window. Personally, I would make mine at 6:00 p.m. and end it at 10:00 p.m., just in time for bed. I also don't like to eat too late, so this seems like the best option. As long as your eating window begins in the early to mid-evening, you can play around with the times.

Choosing Your Food

This is the important one—when it comes to this method you absolutely have to eat the right food during the day, or you may end up gaining weight rather than losing it—not ideal. Below you will find outlined examples of foods you should be incorporating into your diet on a daily basis so that you can be successful.

According to Sadhukhan (2021), here's what your daily routine should look like:

- As a rule, every morning you should head straight to the kitchen and warm up some water. Slice either a lime or lemon in half, add this to the warm water and drink the entire cup. As an added bonus, add a little bit of honey to maximize detoxification of your body, boost your immune system, and improve bowel movements. The lemon helps by balancing your insulin levels and helping reduce body fat, both of which complement your fasting regime.

- Once you have had your water you can think about what you want to eat to start your day. Your best options are foods high in protein to promote satiety as well as fresh fruit. Fruit is packed with fiber, which will also keep your digestive system working optimally and flush out toxins. Some excellent options would be boiled egg whites, or fresh sliced fruits such as strawberries, blueberries, pawpaw, or grapefruit with chia seeds. If you would rather wait until lunch you can always settle for black coffee or green tea to really get your metabolism working.

- For lunch, you'll want to keep things extremely light. Some good options are a cup of yogurt, or a bowl of fresh fruit. One cup of vegetable soup is another excellent, low-calorie option to fill your tummy and provide sustenance.

- In between meals make sure that you are drinking plenty of water.

- Now for the big one—the dinnertime feast! You don't have to order Mcdonalds to really enjoy your food, there are plenty of wholesome delicious options you can choose from that taste even better. And the best part? Each one allows a tasty dessert!

- For your first option, you could prepare a healthy serving of vegetable wheat pasta with one square of tiramisu and a cup of warm milk with some turmeric.

- As a second option, you could have grilled chicken, mashed sweet potato, sauteed vegetables (carrots, green beans, spinach, broccoli, cauliflower), and a cup of warm milk with turmeric. For a tasty post-dinner treat you can enjoy a modest piece of your favorite dark chocolate. Yum!

- Sweet potato, chicken stew, and cauliflower is another tasty option. Nuts, seeds, chocolate, and ice cream are delicious ways to satisfy any post-meal cravings (just don't overdo it, use your discretion).

The combination of protein, complex carbohydrates, and vegetables will ensure all your nutritional requirements are met. Plus, the sweet dessert will satisfy your cravings and keep your taste buds alive and kicking. This is why it is so important to create a balance; you want to make sure that you're not totally depriving yourself of the things you love, as this may cause you to binge later on.

According to Sadhukhan (2021), these are some additional foods that you should be incorporating into your fasting window:

- water, coffee, green tea, or vegetable juice
- eggs (hard-boiled)
- chicken or beef broth
- milk and cheese
- any fruit or vegetable

This next list of foods can be enjoyed during your eating window, but make sure you enjoy them in moderate portions:

- healthy fats such as nuts, seeds, and olive oil

- whole grains in the form of oats, rice, bread, and wheat pasta
- fruits and vegetables
- milk, cheese, and yogurt
- protein such as chicken, fish, beef, and pork

Foods such as fried chicken, cookies, milk chocolate, chips, processed meats, artificial sweeteners, refined carbs, and fizzy sodas should be avoided if possible.

Exercise

Ori Hofmekler, a graduate in Human Sciences and creator of The Warrior Diet, recommends the use of body weight for exercising, rather than using actual weights. Pull-ups, push-ups, and squats are all good examples of this, as well as some HIIT training. HIIT training can be described as short bursts of intense exercise combined with rest and lower-intensity workouts done in between reps. Not only do they keep you super fit, but they're highly effective for weight loss (Hodgkin, 2017). If you're not yet comfortable with this, take your time. Your body is still adapting to this new way of eating and you don't want to place too much stress on it.

Alternate-Day Fasting

There are two ways in which you can practice this form of fasting, with one option offering a more lenient approach. This lenient approach to fasting is known as the modified approach, where you don't have to refrain from eating completely on your fasting days, but you can choose to consume 25% of your typical calorie intake. This makes things a whole lot easier and sustainable, but some people may still choose to refrain from eating completely on their fasting days. Whichever you choose, make sure that you are eating the right foods at the right time to look after your wellbeing, which is exactly what you'll learn here!

Choosing Your Days

Ideally, you should be fasting for one day and then eating normally the next. If you need a recap, I outlined what a typical week would look like in the previous chapter. As you can see, you're alternating between a fasting day and normal eating to keep the balance and reap the benefits. While I mentioned 500 calories as being the aim on these days, you can choose whether you want to eat anything at all on this day or do the modified approach. Personally, I think it's downright crazy to not eat anything at all for multiple days of the week, so I would recommend the modified approach for older women in particular (I'll dive into deeper detail later in this chapter).

That said, if you do decide to try the modified approach, you need to bear in mind that you have to religiously track your calories. If you eat more than 25% of your normal daily intake, then you haven't completed a fast day at all (sadly, this is an easy mistake to make). For this reason, some people do choose to simply fast the entire day to spare themselves the risk and the trouble. I advise that you download a free calorie-tracking app if you choose the moderate approach. This makes things much more convenient and allows you to log your meals throughout the day while the app does the hard part—calculating and memorizing your daily calories!

When choosing your days, you need to plan it so that you are fasting for three days and eating normally for the remaining four; make sure that you allow at least one day's break in between your fasting days for recovery. How you choose to do this is up to you, but you can use the example in the previous chapter as a reference. For now, here is a five-week adjustment schedule you can use to ease your way into alternate-day fasting, according to Kadouch (2020):

- Firstly you need to choose three fasting days per week. So, you could say Monday, Wednesday, and Friday.
- In the first week, start by simply skipping breakfast on all of those fasting days.
- In the second week, you can begin to skip lunch for only one of the fasting days.
- In the third week, try fasting for one entire day or limit your calories to 500 on one of your fasting days.
- In week four you can start to skip lunch on all three fasting days.
- For week five you can fast for all three fasting days, either eating nothing at all or following the modified approach (don't forget your calorie-tracker app)!

Choosing Your Hours

In terms of your hours you just need to make sure you are sticking to your calorie restrictions on your three fasting days and eating normally for the remaining four. The timing of your eating doesn't matter on your non-fasting days, but I personally avoid eating too much too late at night as it can disrupt sleep.

Choosing Your Food

As you know, you are allowed to eat freely on your non-fasting days. On your fasting days; however, you'll need to know how to stick to your calorie limit. That said, I am going to list a few examples below of what 500 calories looks like so that you have a point of reference going forward—here they are!

Option one

- One boiled egg with spinach and mushrooms (120 calories)
- One cup of soup (your choice) (70 calories)
- Steamed broccoli with chicken breast (170 calories)
- Grilled fish with a garden salad (150 calories)

Option two:
- Two pieces of flatbread with low-fat cream cheese (194 calories)
- Chicken and potato leek soup (96 calories)
- Chicken tikka (136 calories)

Option three:
- 1 ½ cups. of low fat-greek yogurt with sliced apricots (68 calories)
- Vegetable soup with croutons and one slice of cheese (140 calories)
- Chicken breast and brown rice with broccoli (170 calories)
- A small bowl of ice cream (130 calories)

Exercise

When it comes to exercise, you can do 15 minutes of light walking on your fasting days, with lightweight training and resistance on your non-fasting days. Don't be afraid to lift weights, as this will help tone and maintain muscle, keeping your metabolism working extra hard when you need it. This is especially important as you grow older.

Hydration

As a general rule, tea, coffee, and water are all permitted on your fasting days. Flavored water should be monitored, as some contain a significant amount of calories. Always watch out for ingredients where you cannot pronounce the name—you can treat that as a red flag (Kadouch, 2020).

In terms of your overnight fasting and spontaneous meal skipping, I've chosen to leave them out of this chapter for one simple reason—they are so incredibly straightforward! As the name suggests, spontaneous meal skipping literally means skipping meals here and there. This may be due to lack of hunger, a full day, or simply not wanting to eat. Overnight fasting on the other hand, simply means that you need to consume your last meal early in the evening and refrain from eating again until the following day, 12 hours after your last meal.

One tip I can give you for overnight fasting is to eat a really well-balanced meal before you go to bed. Lean proteins such as chicken, fish, or even steak are excellent options, as well as broccoli, cauliflower, spinach, potatoes, and other mixed vegetables as sides. If need be, you can indulge in a square or two of dark chocolate to satisfy cravings, but this must all take place before your overnight fasting window begins. I personally recommend fasting from 8:00 p.m. until 8:00 a.m. the following day, but the choice is entirely up to you.

CHAPTER 6

TIPS AND TRICKS FOR ACHIEVING INTERMITTENT FASTING SUCCESS

*Y*ou're finally here—my favorite part of the book and the holy grail of fasting success! If you're going to succeed on this incredible journey, then you'll need to equip yourself with all the fasting know-how available, which is exactly where this chapter comes in. Let's dive in!

What Can I Expect When Starting to Fast?

The best way to succeed is by managing your expectations and being prepared! It's only natural that your body will feel different when making a change, so it's not something to worry about. When you first start to fast, the most obvious thing that you can expect is hunger. While it may be tough to fight your cravings in the beginning, you'll find that your hunger naturally dissipates after resisting your initial urges. Another common side effect is irritability—I'm sure we can all relate to the term, 'hangry' when we haven't eaten and the cravings make us super cranky (we've all been there at some point)!

You may feel slightly sluggish and fatigued in your adjustment stage, but this will also fade as your body adapts. All that said, most healthy individuals don't have any major side effects when they begin fasting, so you definitely shouldn't panic.

How Do I Know I'm Fasting Correctly?

Fasting is about so much more than simply abstaining from food for a specified period of time. A successful fast is composed of a variety of success indicators that not only benefit your weight loss goals, but your mental clarity, peace of mind, and energy levels. There are six primary criteria to determine a successful fast, which I will summarize below for you:

- You successfully complete a fast during the specified time frame that you set for yourself.

- You are aware of your fasting goals before you begin your fast, and you achieve them at the end.

- Besides fasting, you make an effort to improve other aspects of your life in conjunction with fasting, rather than seeing fasting as a fix-all approach.

- You fast for a variety of health-related reasons, including mental clarity, spirituality, and disease prevention (your goal should not focus solely on weight loss).

- You eat wholesome, nutrient-dense foods even after your fast is complete.

- You are able to easily transition in and out of your fast.

- You maintain your weight loss even after you stop fasting.

Looking at the above-mentioned points, you can see that fasting is changing your lifestyle holistically, as well as spiritually, mentally, physically, and emotionally. Too many women view fasting as a "quick fix" to their unhealthy relationship with food, and this simply isn't the case. Fasting should be done properly and for the right reasons—if you find that you are continuously breaking your fast, you may want to try a different method for weight loss ("12 Tips to Achieve Fasting Success," 2021).

Keep trying until you find what works for you. It's all part of the journey!

17 Key Tips for Fasting Success

Master Self-Control

While this may seem obvious, this is one of the most critical aspects of intermittent fasting. It goes without saying that you are going to be hungry, and the first few hours into your fast are always the hardest. That leftover piece of pie is going to be calling your name, as well as that pack of muffins in your cupboard. These cravings are perfectly normal, and it doesn't mean that you're not cut out for this journey. What truly defines your willpower is the ability to say no and push through these momentary cravings. Remember, there is a big difference between your body *wanting* food and actually *needing* food, and you'll be able to tell if you watch out for the symptoms. During a normal 12-16 hour fast, it's highly unlikely that you're going to experience any severe indications of hunger. Signs that your body desperately needs calories are nausea, dizziness, and chills. Simply feeling peckish or experiencing a rumbling in your stomach is a temporary feeling and will go away once you push through the initial cravings.

Watch Your Carbs

While I am certainly not the type of person to bash carbs (in fact, I believe the *right* types of carbs are really important in any diet), you need to make sure that you are eating healthy, complex carbs such as the low-GI variety, whole grains, whole wheat, quinoa, and barley. If you indulge in simple carbs such as white bread, cakes, and white rice, your body will experience intense spikes and crashes in insulin and blood sugar, and this will wreak havoc on your cravings. You'll find yourself running to the cupboard in a starved frenzy for sugar before you know it, and all your hard work will be in vain!

Lay Out Your Objectives

First things first, you need to clearly define your objectives for starting this new journey. You need to ask yourself why you are doing this and what you hope to achieve so that you can set reminders for motivation along the way. Start by investing in a cute new journal; open up a fresh, blank page and start writing. You can do it in a list style or you can simply write what comes to mind, but make sure you are clear about what you hope to achieve. This will be your point of reference going forward, especially when you are feeling discouraged or anxious about why you're doing this ("12 Tips to Achieve Fasting Success," 2021).

For example, this is what your list of objectives could look like:

- To achieve a healthier relationship with food
- Achieve a healthy weight
- Live a longer, healthier life
- Prevent disease
- To be more mindful about food rather than eating for the sake of eating
- To detox and cleanse toxins from many years of bad eating habits

Log all of these into your book and keep them aside for reference if need be. Every time you feel tempted to cheat, refer back to this list to remind yourself why it is so important to persevere and succeed.

Keep Fasting Periods Short to Begin With

As you know by now, there are several methods of fasting that each have the same goal. That said, you can choose how long you choose to fast—whether you choose 24 hours or only 12, you do what feels most comfortable. Regardless of how long you intend to fast, it's really important that you start off slowly. Start off by simply skipping a meal here and there, and see how you feel. After one week you can attempt to fast for 12-14 hours a few days per week, as you would with the crescendo approach. Gradually, you can advance your fasting duration as your body adapts (West, 2019). Remember, slow and steady wins the race!

Prepare Yourself Mentally

This one is super important—you have to be in the right headspace before striving to complete a fast! You need to begin your fast with the intention to succeed, otherwise, you'll quickly create a mental block. Read through your list of goals, and take the time to read blogs written by others who have taken a similar path. You can find some really motivational stories written by others that can help prepare you for the journey ahead, and understand that you're not alone ("12 Tips to Achieve Fasting Success," 2021).

Feel free to have your favorite meal or treat before you begin your fast, as this will minimize any cravings later on in the process. You can also watch Youtube videos of others where they log their cravings, emotions, and general experiences during the fasting process. If you feel any unexpected side effects, it may make you feel better if other people have experienced them too and persevered!

Take Supplements

While you should be okay if you're eating wholesome, nutrient-rich foods during your non-fasting days, it is possible for long-term fasters to be deficient in certain nutrients. Women over the age of 50 need to be particularly careful about their calcium intake, as well as selenium, magnesium, folate, iron, and vitamins B6, B12, and D. As a precaution, it is recommended that you take daily supplements to ensure strong bones, joints, and various other bodily functions (West, 2019).

Listen to Your Body

I cannot stress enough the importance of listening to your body! While it is true that you need to motivate yourself and persevere, there's a difference between craving chocolate and feeling genuinely weak, dizzy, and lightheaded from not eating. Additional warning signs are headaches, intense fatigue, feeling cold, anxious, and the inability to focus on a task. These are all signs that your body seriously needs fuel and you shouldn't ignore them. While it's perfectly normal to feel some of these symptoms in a milder form when you first start fasting, prolonged, severe symptoms indicate that fasting may not be the best option for you.

Sleep, Sleep, Sleep

One key component of looking after yourself is making sure that you are getting enough sleep. Most people need between seven to nine hours of sleep per night, with older people needing slightly less (around six to seven hours). That said, everyone is different. You will generally know how many hours you need to function properly, so you need to do your best to stick to these. The reason this is so important is that lack of sleep wreaks havoc with your ghrelin and leptin levels which control your hunger. When you are sleep-deprived, they are all out of whack and this causes you to feel hungry—even when you're not.

The combination of hunger and exhaustion will result in you eating constantly throughout the day to keep going, and this will inevitably cause weight gain. Getting sufficient sleep will help you function at your best and regulate your hormones so that you don't experience cravings.

Don't Overeat When Breaking Your Fast

Trust me, *I get it*—you're going to be absolutely ravenous when you near the end of your fast, naturally! That said, this is no excuse to binge eat pizza, burgers, and chips. What your body needs is a moderate portion of whole, unprocessed foods such as protein, complex carbs, and vegetables. Plus, your stomach will have shrunk slightly during your fast, so you'll likely feel full surprisingly quickly once you do break your fast. The last thing you want to feel is bloated and uncomfortably full, especially considering all the hard work and effort you put into your fast. Always remember to focus more on the *quality* of foods rather than the *quantity*—that way you can't go wrong!

Don't Panic

Your mind is an exceptionally powerful thing, and you can harness this power for the positive or negative. Many people refuse to fast because they claim that they absolutely *have to* eat all the time and they have headaches or dizziness if they don't, or they come up with a myriad of other excuses as to why they are different and cannot fast. The truth is, a human with normal body weight can actually survive for approximately 40 days without food. So, claiming that you're starving after one day without food sounds pretty ridiculous.

Yes, it's going to be difficult and you'll need a lot of willpower, but it's highly unlikely that you're putting your body through any harm. In fact, 90% of hunger cues are in the mind, meaning you're not actually feeling true hunger. Remember, the majority of your fears come from the mind, and it's up to you to control them so that you can achieve your goals ("12 Tips to Achieve Fasting Success," 2021).

Find Calming Yet Stimulating Activities

If you find your mind wandering toward the idea of food while fasting, you need to find an activity that is healthy, stimulating, and not overly strenuous. Meditation is an excellent way to not only find inner peace but to train your mind not to wander and focus on healthy, calming thoughts. Yoga is another excellent option, as well as walking, listening to music, or having a bath (West, 2019).

The key is to find a go-to activity that you can turn to when you feel the urge to cheat. Personally, I find that taking my dog for a walk when I have the urge to binge is an excellent distraction. I grab a bottle of water and sip it throughout my walk, and take the uphill climb back home. By the time I'm back I feel alive and positive and the need to snack on unnecessary things has vanished.

Team Up

While this may appear contradictory to the point mentioned above, if you can find someone who genuinely supports you, and even better, wants to embark on this journey together, then that's great. Having someone join you in your fast will help give you that extra push on your hardest days and motivate you to share good news when you succeed. You can also empathize and share experiences, assuring you that you're not alone in what you're feeling.

It can also be difficult to follow a fasting schedule and healthier eating when your friends and family aren't doing the same. Of course, there is no need for your family to fast with you if they don't want to, but simply having them eat healthier meals along with you removes the temptation of watching friends and family eat junk while you remain disciplined.

Understand Your Emotions

During your fasting journey, you are going to experience a whole range of emotions, including frustration, disappointment, self-criticism, cravings, and irritation. Although this sounds daunting, you need to embrace these emotions as part of the journey! Start by identifying as many as you can and ask yourself why you are feeling these emotions, then you can work through them and take control.

If you're feeling stressed or sad, acknowledge those emotions and try to pinpoint where they came from and what can be done to rectify them besides eating to avoid the problem. While this isn't always the easiest thing to do, it can be done with some practice and consistency.

Eat Slowly and Often During Your Eating Window

When you fast for long hours it's imperative that you make sure you are receiving enough nutrients. Since you're compressing your calorie consumption into a significantly smaller eating window, you should make sure that you are eating smaller meals throughout the day to balance sugar levels and take in nutrients. Make sure that you are eating a variety of foods that include protein, carbs, vegetables, and fruits so that you don't miss out on important vitamins and minerals ("A Fasting Diet Shouldn't

Turn You Into a Hangry Betch—Here's How to Do it Right," 2021).

Prepare Meals in Advance

As I'm sure you already know, life can get really crazy sometimes. Unfortunately, sometimes we drop the ball when things get too busy, and this includes healthy eating. Have you ever ordered that greasy takeout at work simply because you are starving and it's cheap, quick, and easy? You can avoid this mistake by preparing healthy, balanced meals the night before or simply cooking a little extra dinner to take to work. Even if your colleagues are tempting you into chipping in for some pizza, you're far less likely to take the bait if you've got a packed lunch in the fridge!

Further in this book I've included an extensive recipe collection with meals you can share with the family or simply freeze and store in the fridge, making meal prepping super easy and convenient.

Protein is Your Friend

When it comes to *any* diet, protein should form a staple part of your dietary intake. Why? Because protein is really good for your body, and I'll list a few of the key benefits below ("Why is Protein Important in Your Diet," 2021).

- As women grow older, they naturally lose more muscle. Protein helps to build and maintain muscle, as well as hair, skin, nails, cartilage, and bones.

- Your body uses protein to repair muscle tissue.

- As women grow older their hormones tend to wreak havoc with them. Protein can help to manage and regulate hormones to minimize complications.

- Your red blood cells require protein to transport oxygen throughout the body, which (obviously), requires a healthy intake of protein.

- 50% of the protein you consume is converted into digestive enzymes which is vital for the healthy functioning of your system.

As a rule, you should aim to eat at least 30% protein when filling up your plate. Foods high in protein include beans, fish, poultry, fresh spinach, eggs, yogurt, pork, and cheese. You can even purchase protein shakes that are jam-packed with additional minerals and vitamins that your body needs ("Why is Protein Important in Your Diet," 2021).

How to Avoid Emotional Eating

We've all been there—your boss has been on your case all day, the kids are screaming, and your bank just called to remind you that your repayments are overdue. How does all of this make you feel? Stressed as hell! For some, they are able to acknowledge and process their emotions and handle them appropriately. For others, they bottle things up and turn to food as a source of comfort. Food is seen as a way to suppress emotions and self-soothe in an attempt to run away from your problems, but this only creates a much bigger one—an unhealthy relationship with food.

As studies have shown, women are far more susceptible to emotional eating than men, which is why it is so important that this problem is addressed. Sadly, women get stuck in a vicious cycle of binging, guilt, and shame, which leads them to eat more. This is why it is important to learn to eat mindfully, as this is the key to avoiding emotional eating. When this cycle gets out of hand, the person struggles to differentiate between true hunger and emotions, which brings me to my next point (Legg, 2018).

How Do I Differentiate Between True Hunger and Emotional Hunger?

When it comes to emotional hunger, the feeling of hunger will be sudden and unexpected. You'll likely have a craving for a very specific food, and your mind will fixate on this. When eating, you may also struggle to feel when you are full, leading you to eat uncontrollably and feel shame and guilt. True hunger, on the other hand, will come about gradually, and you'll have a craving for all types of foods. This will help you know when you are full and follow the cue to stop eating, so you don't have any unhealthy feelings of guilt or shame once you have completed the meal (Legg, 2018).

As a rule of thumb, I always picture the idea of an apple in my mind. If I feel the urge to eat it, then I know I am genuinely hungry. If not, then I know I'm just craving junk for the sake of eating! If you know that you're losing the battle, you need to stop, breathe, and ask yourself why you are feeling these emotions. Ask yourself what you are feeling—are you sad? If so, why? Write your feelings down if you need to and acknowledge them.

Try and come up with small actions you can do now to work toward solving the problem, rather than turning to food. Remind yourself how you felt the last time you overindulged your feelings through food and why you don't want to feel that way again. As I mentioned earlier, going for walks, meditating, or reading a book are much healthier coping mechanisms. When you feel the urge to binge, make the decision to do something else and act on it immediately before your brain tries to stop you.

Another preventative measure is throwing out any triggering foods that you know can cause a binge. Cookies, chips, and cupcakes are all temptations that are going to play on your mind. If you don't have the heart to throw out the junk, at least keep it out of sight and out of mind. If you have a jar of cookies sitting on your kitchen counter, you're asking for trouble! You can even place these triggering foods somewhere out of reach so that it's simply not worth the effort to try and obtain them.

Most importantly, simply stocking your fridge and pantry with whole, unprocessed foods means that you will have no choice but to eat what's there. Another tip that works for me is dishing up smaller portions for myself before I head to the couch or the table. If you grab the entire packet of food, you're more likely to mindlessly finish the whole thing, compared to dishing out a smaller portion and putting the rest away.

You can also tell a loved one about your struggles and turn to them for support when you're feeling anxious, sad, or depressed. A quick phone call to a loved one can really lift your spirits, as well as joining a support group with other like-minded people. Remember, you're not alone! Lastly, you owe it to yourself to speak to yourself kindly—positive self-talk is so important. If you can't say your thoughts about yourself out loud to others, then you should change your way of thinking. Treat yourself with bubble baths, facials, and lunches, and be a little kinder to your body.

What About Binge Eating?

Binge eating and emotional eating are usually connected, and the individual finds it incredibly difficult to stop eating once they have started. The best way to combat this is by practicing mindful eating, meaning that you are acknowledging your senses as you consume your meal. For example, instead of grabbing a meal or packet of chips and heading for the couch and TV, take your meal and eat it at a table. When you distract your mind with TV or other stimulating activities, you're no longer paying attention to your signals of fullness or hunger. Instead, you're simply eating for the sake of eating and this results in you eating too much and gaining weight.

I'm sure you can recall a time when you were watching a good movie with a large packet of crisps or popcorn, and you were horrified to find that you had finished the entire bag without even realizing it! This is because you were not eating to appreciate the taste, texture, and pleasure of the food, but you were simply eating for the sake of it. Always practice mindful eating!

How to Avoid Fasting Side Effects

When it comes to the side effects of fasting, many of the most common ones are caused by simple mistakes that are easily avoided. Below I am going to list some of the most common side effects and how you can avoid making the same mistakes.

Diarrhea

Some people report experiencing diarrhea when they first begin to fast. There are two possible reasons for this; namely your body flushing out excess fluids and salts, and surprisingly, breaking your fast! When you finally break your fast, your GI tract kicks back into motion and this can result in you rushing to the bathroom; so, it's not the act of fasting itself. Drinking lots of caffeine during your fast may also trigger an upset stomach, so keep an eye on that. Diarrhea may also be a result of the foods you are eating, with milk, refined carbohydrates, and legumes being common culprits. While legumes are really good for you and highly recommended, their high fiber content may be causing diarrhea (Lederer, 2020).

In an attempt to evade all of this, avoid caffeinated beverages and sweeteners, and drink plenty of water if you have already had an upset stomach. Cucumber water and bone broth are also excellent remedies for diarrhea (Lederer, 2020).

Bad Breath

Okay, so this probably isn't the most appealing side effect of fasting, but it has been reported by some. If you're wondering what causes this, it's due to a lack of saliva in the mouth and an increase in acetone in the breath. The acetone is a by-product which comes from the increase in fat-burning for fuel. So, there will be much higher levels of acetone in your blood and breath, resulting in an unpleasant odor (Kubala, 2021). The best way to combat this is by investing in some chewing gum or breath mints, and keeping your distance! That said, I've fasted for years and I've never had any comments or problems in this regard, but then again, my partner may be a good liar!

Sleep Changes

Some people find that fasting interferes with their ability to fall asleep normally. Unfortunately, this is one of the more common side effects of fasting, so it's best to prepare yourself. That said, if you've ever tried to go to bed with an empty stomach, you'll know how difficult it can be. One 2020 study found that 15% of the 1,422 participants practicing fasting experienced problems related to falling and staying asleep, and this seemed to be the prominent side effect related to fasting (Kubala, 2021).

The best thing you can do to avoid this is to try and eliminate habits that can contribute to sleep disturbances. Alcohol, cigarettes, blue light from TV and computers, and too much caffeine too late in the afternoon can all contribute to insomnia. You can also try and time your meals so that you don't eat too late but not too early either (around 7:00 p.m. is ideal). If you eat too late, your body may keep you awake as it's so busy trying to digest the food. On the other hand, if you eat too early, you'll be hungry just before bedtime and that can keep you up too (Kubala, 2021).

Fatigue

Now, this is a common problem. Many people report feeling sluggish during the first few days of fasting, and this is perfectly normal; however, this isn't ideal if you have a busy lifestyle and have tasks to complete that require energy. One of the many myths surrounding IF is that you should engage in minimal exercise while you fast, which simply isn't true. Your body needs exercise in order to shift your body into fat-burning mode and ramp up energy levels. When you feel tired, this is your body's way of indicating that carbohydrate stores are depleting, and your body is trying to preserve as much energy as possible (Lederer, 2020).

In order to counteract this you need to engage in some form of exercise to deplete these stores and shift your body into fat burning mode. Something as simple as a walk or yoga will do, and you will immediately notice an improvement in your energy levels. Light weight resistance training is also a good option, as it works with fasting to promote muscle growth. This is because fasting prompts the body to release more human growth hormone which helps build and maintain muscle, so training compliments this effect (Lederer, 2020). So, next time you're feeling tired, get up and move!

No Results

As disappointing and demotivating as this is, some women find that they simply aren't seeing results despite following the correct fasting methods. One common mistake that I personally have made (along with many other women) is adding full-fat milk and sugar to my coffee. Did you know that one cup of coffee with whole milk and two sugars can pack nearly 100 calories?

Now, imagine you're drinking three to four cups a day. Not only are you breaking your fast, but you're taking in hundreds of empty calories every day, which can build up very quickly. Sadly, that dash of milk and sugar will cause you to break the fast by increasing sugar and insulin levels, which counteracts the benefits of fasting. Rather, stick to black coffee and tea, and avoid diet sodas or anything with artificial sweeteners, as these will break your fast too (Lederer, 2020).

Headaches

That pesky headache that women complain about may not be for the reasons you think—fasting headaches may be the result of a lack of sodium. Strangely, salt has been demonized in the past as a health threat when consumed in excess; however, studies have shown that people who eat more salt are less susceptible to cardiovascular disease (Lederer, 2020). Plus, your body will indicate to you that you've had enough salt by killing cravings, whereas the same cannot be said for sugar—your body just craves more!

In fact, Dr. Jason Fung, an endocrinologist, found that the majority of IF side effects stem from a salt deficiency, including headaches and fatigue. So, don't be afraid to sprinkle some salt over your meals where needed, and opt for Pink Himalayan salt as it is in a more natural form and won't contain anti-caking agents, which are powdered ingredients commonly added to confectionaries to prevent lumps. Certain studies indicate that anti-caking agents may degrade the vitamins and minerals in foods, which is why some people believe that they should be avoided (Lederer, 2020).

Another reason for fasting headaches could be due to hypoglycemia, which is associated with the changes in glucose levels that take place when you fast. Not every person experiences this, as this appears to be more of a genetic predisposition; however, it is believed that the changes in glucose cause the pain receptors in the brain to activate; thus, causing these headaches to occur. That said, not every expert agrees with this theory, and believes that there are other causes besides glucose (Doherty, 2020).

Another more likely cause of fasting headaches is simply due to dehydration. This, combined with the stress signals in the body when in a fasted state, may be a viable explanation for why fasting headaches occur. So, the best thing that you can do is drink plenty of water throughout the day and see if that makes any difference in how you feel. That said, fasting headaches are not considered to be common side effects, so don't worry too much about this (Doherty, 2020).

How Do I Track My Progress?

If you're going to get anywhere with fasting, you'll need to have some method of keeping track of your daily food intake, eating windows, and fasting periods. With so much going on in life, it can be difficult to keep track of even the smallest of things, so you'll definitely need a helping hand when it comes to this!

The good news is that there are several apps you can download to help you keep track of your progress. Since they're so sophisticated you do have to pay for them, but some of them are extremely affordable with prices as low as $2.99. According to Cohen (2020), some of the best options for tracking your progress are:

- Window
- Vora
- FastHabit
- Fastient
- LIFE Fasting Tracker
- BodyFast
- Zero
- Fastic (this one won't cost you a cent for the basic version, but you have the option to pay for an upgrade).

With these apps, you have the option to keep a diary of your thoughts, track your weight, sleep, and personalized plans, as well as daily progress alerts. These apps make your life a whole lot easier by acting as a portable, interactive logbook that you can carry around with you wherever you go—extremely convenient!

If you find that you're still not losing weight and you've tried absolutely everything in terms of diet and exercise, then it may be a good idea to see your healthcare practitioner and get an examination. It is not uncommon for older women to have hypothyroidism or polycystic ovarian syndrome and these can make it extremely difficult to lose weight (Kubala, 2019). If you consistently experience fatigue, swelling, constipation, and dry skin, then you may want to get checked out by a professional (please don't take this as a diagnosis, your doctor needs to examine you).

Once you find out the underlying cause of your frustrating lack of progress, you'll be able to move forward with a solution provided by your doctor. And the best part? You can *finally* stop beating yourself up!

How to Maintain Intermittent Fasting

When it comes to maintenance, I can only stress two things—sustainability and lifestyle. I mentioned earlier in this book that fasting should not be viewed as a quick fix but rather as a lifestyle choice. You shouldn't view fasting as something you do to quickly shed some pounds and then revert back to eating junk. Remember I mentioned earlier in this chapter about being in the right headspace before you begin fasting? This is so important for the maintenance of the diet and success. You need to alter your mindset to enjoy eating healthy, wholesome foods and view fasting in a more holistic manner. In other words, fasting is not a diet, but rather a lifestyle that can improve many aspects of your mental and physical health.

You don't have to fast every day for the rest of your life, but you can set aside certain days of the week when you feel your body needs it most. What you do need to keep constant, however, are the foods you eat. You need to find healthy foods that you enjoy so that eating them doesn't feel like a punishment or chore. For me, hummus and cucumber sticks are my new addiction and they're incredibly healthy and delicious. Learning to spice up simple, healthy meals such as chicken and vegetables can also turn a less-exciting meal into a really tasty one.

Later in this book, you'll find a whole bunch of healthy, delicious recipes that you can try out to excite your taste buds and get you motivated to prepare new, healthy dishes. Once you train your body to enjoy wholesome, unprocessed foods, you'll find that your body no longer craves junk food. As long as you incorporate some light exercise and whole foods into your lifestyle, you won't gain back the weight you've lost.

Foods to Eat While Fasting

When it comes to fasting there are certain foods that you should set as your go-to options and others that should be avoided. Foods that you should be regularly enjoying should be fiber-rich, full of vitamins and minerals, antioxidants, and low-GI. This means you're getting the best bang for your buck with every mouthful and you're nourishing your body as you eat. That said, here are some of your best go-to options:

- lentils
- potatoes
- berries (raspberries, strawberries, blackberries, blueberries)

- fresh salmon
- hummus
- water, coffee, or tea
- minimally processed grains
- soybeans
- smoothies
- red wine
- nuts
- papaya
- avocados
- cruciferous vegetables
- probiotics

Foods to Avoid While Fasting

Most of the options listed below should be avoided naturally, as they're high in sodium, unhealthy fats, cholesterol, and sugar. When it comes to fasting, you should be especially wary of these foods and avoid them when you can. Here are your fasting don'ts:

- all processed foods such as ham, bacon, cakes, biscuits, pies, sausage links, and chips
- simple carbs such as white bread and rice
- sweetened fruit juice
- sweets
- greasy fast foods
- energy drinks and sugary sodas

While it's okay to enjoy these foods as a treat once in a while, they definitely shouldn't make up the majority of your diet. As tasty as they are, you're not doing your body or your health any favors!

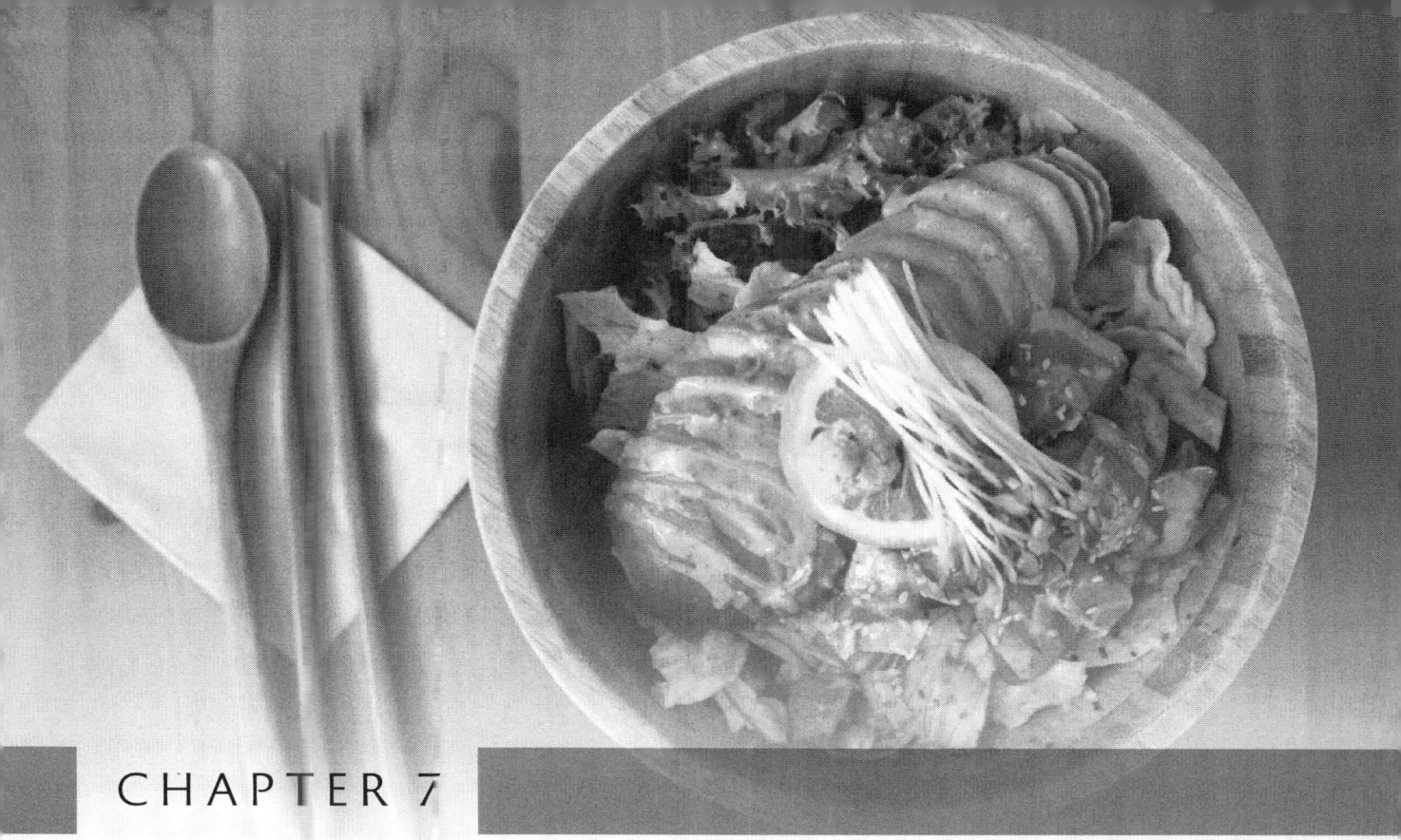

CHAPTER 7

40 INTERMITTENT FASTING QUALITY RECIPES FOR WEIGHT LOSS AND ANTI-AGING

You've done it—you've reached the end of this book (well, almost)! Now that you know all the tips and tricks, it's time to dive into what really matters, and that's how you are going to prepare your meals. In this chapter, you will find a variety of tasty, healthy recipes that are packed with anti-aging antioxidants and all the nutrients you'll need to lose weight and make it through your fasts. The foods you eat play an integral role in the appearance of your skin, hair bones, and joints, which is why it is so important that you nourish your body with the right meals (Winn, 2021). Let's get started!

ORANGE AND APRICOT QUINOA

Cooking Time: 20 minutes

If you choose to time your fast so that you include breakfast, then this is the perfect option! Packed with fiber, vitamin C, and healthy complex carbs, this super-healthy breakfast promotes anti-aging, satiety, and will provide you with sustainable energy throughout the day. The ingredients can also help ward off cancer, heart problems, and boosts skin and brain health (Mazzoni, 2021). Dig in!

Why We Love it

Nutrition facts

Servings: 1

Carbs: 55 g

Protein: 8 g

Fat: 6 g

Net carbs: 34 g

Calorie count per serving: 480

Ingredients

- ½ cup quinoa
- 1 pinch cinnamon
- 4 dried and chopped apricots
- 1 tbsp hazelnuts
- grated orange zest
- fresh orange juice

Instructions

1. Grab a saucepan and prepare the quinoa as the package instructs, but make sure that you replace half of the water with fresh orange juice.
2. Next, toss in one generous pinch of cinnamon.
3. Once the quinoa is cooked, remove it from the pan and use a fork to fluff the quinoa.
4. Toss in the sliced apricot and the hazelnuts.
5. To finish, decorate the dish with the grated orange zest and enjoy!

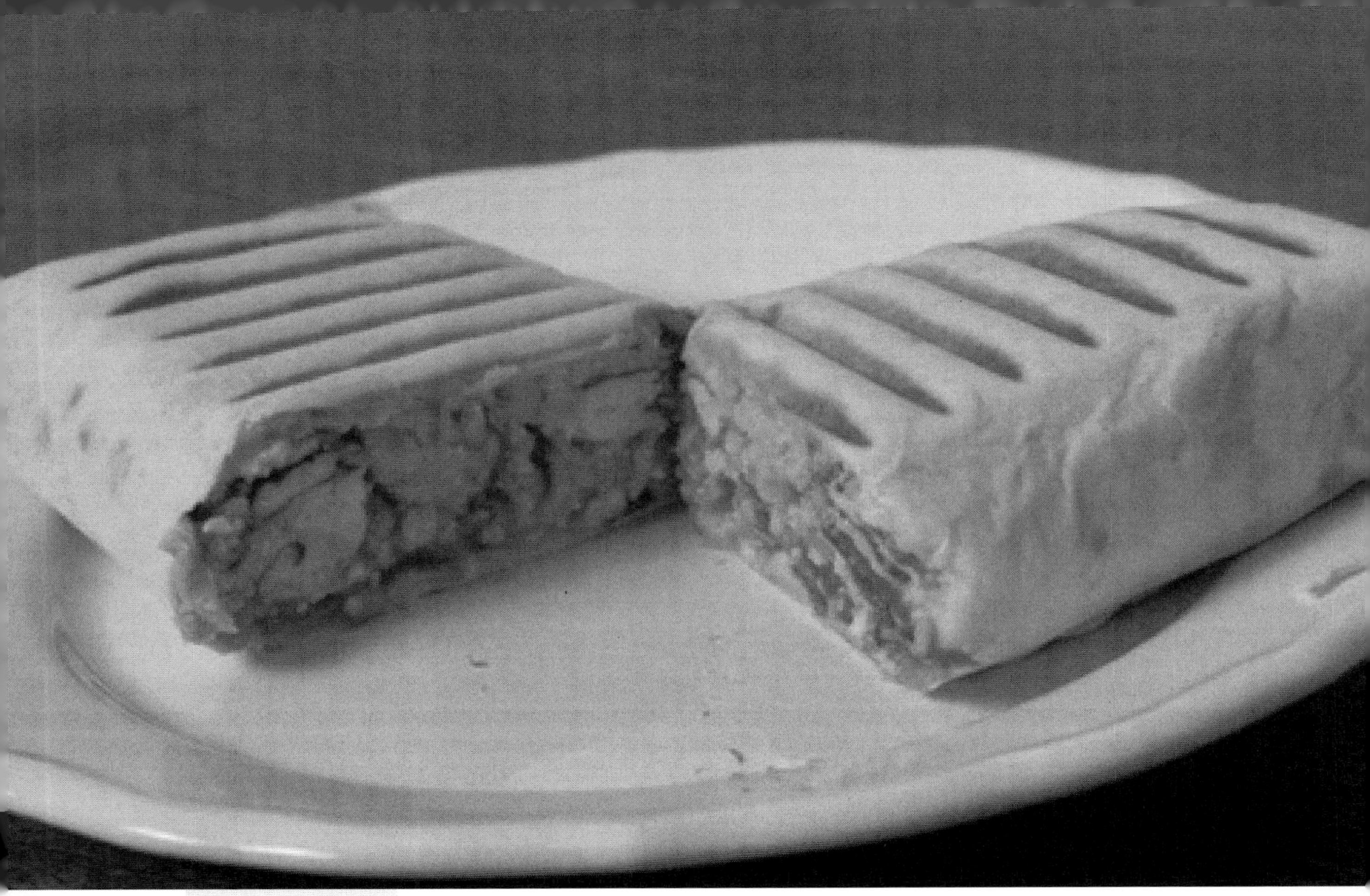

SUPER HEALTHY
BREAKFAST BURRITO

Cooking time: 38 minutes

Why We Love it

If you plan to start your fast later on in the day, then this is the perfect morning option. It's got all the vitamins and minerals you need, with enough carbs, healthy fats, and protein to carry you through your upcoming fast.

Nutrition facts

Servings: 1
Carbs: 59.4 g
Protein: 23 g

Fat: 20 g
Net carbs: 51 g
Calorie count per serving: 460

Ingredients

- 4 eggs
- 4 egg whites
- ¼ tsp chili flakes
- 2 tsp canola oil
- ½ small red onion (chopped)
- 1 cup diced red bell pepper
- salt and pepper to taste
- ¼ cup salsa
- ⅓ cup shredded cheese
- 1 avocado (small)
- hot sauce of choice (optional)
- 1 large tomato
- 1 cup black beans (drained)
- 4 burrito-sized whole wheat tortillas
- ¼ cup sour cream or Greek yogurt (low-fat)

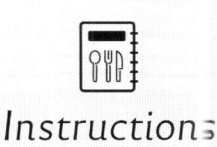
Instructions

1. Taking a large nonstick skillet, heat the pan and all of the canola oil on a medium-high heat.
2. For the next eight minutes, cook the onions and peppers until the onions are tender and the peppers are slightly charred.
3. Next, toss in the chili flakes and black beans; leave them to cook for a further three minutes. Once done, you can sprinkle some salt and pepper for flavor.
4. Next, combine the eggs and egg whites with the cheese in a separate bowl.
5. Spray the skillet with cooking spray and set it over medium heat, then add the eggs and turn the heat down slightly.
6. Scramble the eggs thoroughly and cook for three minutes.
7. Spread the tortillas evenly with the sour cream and throw in some salsa, then add ¼ of the mixture of black beans.
8. Slice the avocado, remove the seed and skin, and set aside.
9. Next, add ¼ of the scrambled eggs, ¼ avocado, and the diced tomato. If you want, you can add some hot sauce for extra flavor.
10. Finally, roll up the burrito and take a bite!

SAVORY STEEL CUT MEAL

Cooking time: 35 minutes

While this meal may seem a little unconventional, this is one of the best meals you can eat as it's quick, packed with protein, and will keep you going throughout the day! You can have this for breakfast, lunch, or dinner—making it perfectly versatile and ideal for anyone's fasting schedule.

Why We Love it

Nutrition facts

Servings: 1

Carbs: 29.8 g

Protein: 13.7 g

Fat: 13.4 g

Net carbs: 27 g

Calorie count per serving: 295

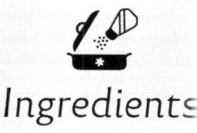
Ingredients

- 1 cup of steel-cut oats
- 3 cups of water
- 1 cup of milk (almond, dairy, or coconut, it is up to you)
- 1 tbsp olive oil or unsalted butter
- freshly ground black pepper to taste
- ¼ tsp salt
- grated cheese of choice
- sauteed vegetables of choice (leafy greens are recommended such as kale and spinach)
- roasted nuts of choice or seeds (optional)
- eggs of choice (scrambled, poached, fried)

Instructions

1. In a large pan, mix together the milk and water and bring to a simmer over medium heat.
2. While you wait, you can start by warming a large skillet and melting the butter.
3. Once the butter has heated you can toss the steel cut oats into the skillet and stir for two minutes until the oats turn a golden hue.
4. Next, add the cooked oats to the saucepan with milk and water and turn the heat down slightly to medium-low.
5. Leave the mixture to cook for approximately 25 minutes and stir frequently until the mixture has thickened.
6. Now it's time to stir in the flavor! Toss in some salt and stir frequently for ten minutes, making sure it doesn't burn by turning down the heat. After ten minutes you will notice the oatmeal is much thicker and creamier.
7. Finally, remove the oatmeal from the heat and allow it to cool for five minutes. You can add any toppings from the list that you wish to add once it has cooled, and season with additional spices if required.
8. Serve your delicious savory oatmeal into a bowl and dig in!

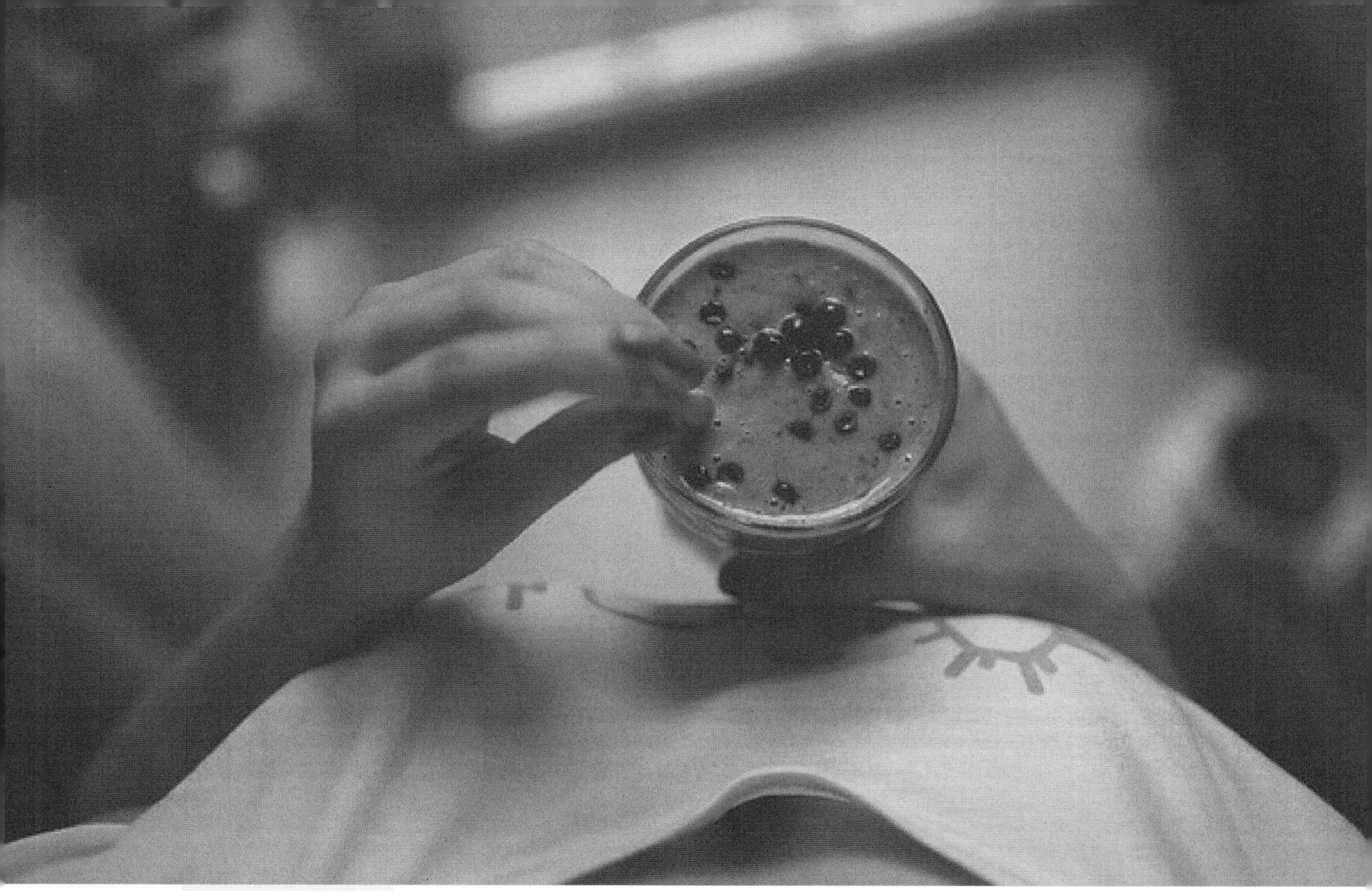

POMEGRANATE YOGURT

Cooking time: 2 minutes

Why We Love it

This next recipe is exceptionally easy to prepare, and will only take a few minutes of your time. I love this option as it's super healthy and tasty, and it's the perfect snack to keep you going, especially if you're following the 5:2 method or The Warrior Diet and need something light to snack on during fasting days. It's also packed with anti-aging properties and healthy fats, so you'll definitely want to incorporate this into your routine.

Nutrition facts

Servings: 1
Carbs: 19 g
Protein: 5 g
Fat: 0g
Net carbs: 12 g
Calorie count per serving: 160

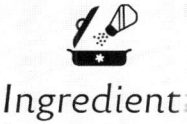

Ingredients

- 1 tbsp sunflower seeds (raw)
- ¾ cup Greek yogurt
- 1 oz 100% pomegranate juice

Instructions

1. Simply spoon the yogurt into a small bowl and pour in the pomegranate juice, mixing gently until combined.
2. Sprinkle some sunflower seeds on the top and dig in!

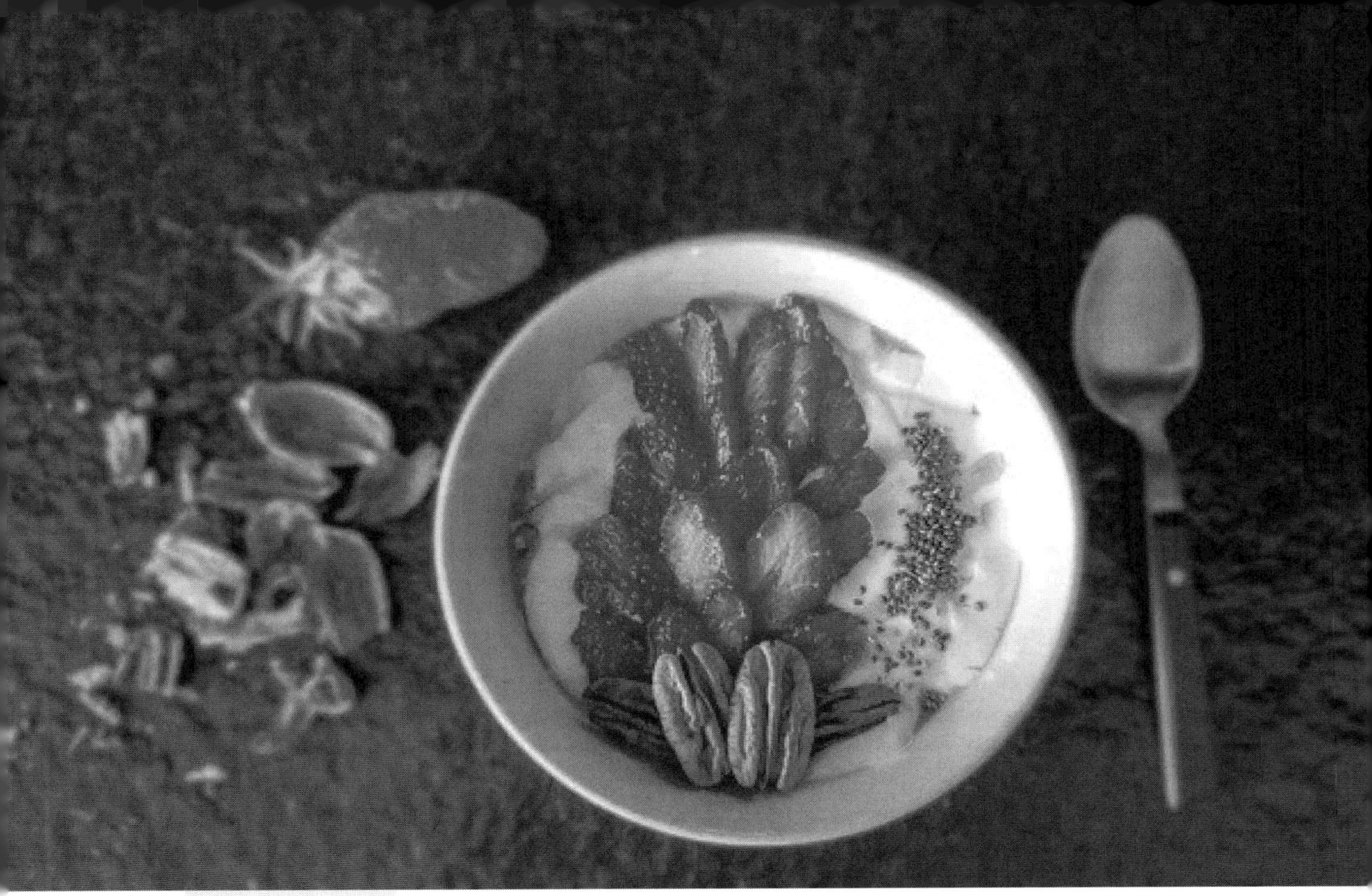

ACAI BREAKFAST BOWL

Cooking time: 5 minutes

Why We Love it

This super-healthy breakfast option is quick to prepare and contains every vitamin and mineral that you could ever need to power through the day with vitality. If there ever was a fountain of youth in a bowl, then you're looking right at it!

Nutrition facts

Servings: 1
Carbs: 65 g
Protein: 9 g
Fat 37 g
Net carbs: 35 g
Calorie count per serving: 211

Ingredients

- 1 packet of acai berries (frozen)
- ¼ cup granola (gluten-free)
- ¼ cup blueberries (frozen)
- 1 banana (frozen)
- 1 tbsp chia seeds
- ½ cup almond milk
- 1 handful strawberries
- 1 handful raspberries
- 1 tbsp coconut (shredded)

Instructions

1. Start by combining the banana, blueberries, acai, and almond milk into a blender and mix until smooth, thick, and creamy.
2. Sprinkle some chia seeds, strawberries, granola, coconut, and berries on top.
3. Enjoy!

BANANA FLAX
BREAKFAST MUFFINS

Cooking time: 30 minutes

These delicious little babies are the perfect on-the-go snack to provide you with plenty of fiber and energy. With flaxseed being one of the main ingredients, you're getting a good dose of omega 3's and protein in a very small package.

Why We Love it

Nutrition facts

Servings: 12 muffins

Carbs: 48 g

Protein: 5 g

Fat: 7 g

Net carbs: 43 g

Calorie count per serving: 252

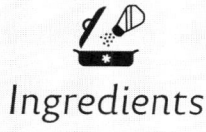
Ingredients

- 4 bananas
- ¼ cup flaxseed meal
- ¼ cup canola oil
- 2 cups bran cereal
- 1 cup of buttermilk (low-fat)
- 1 egg (large)
- ¼ tsp salt
- ¼ tsp nutmeg (ground)
- ½ tsp baking soda
- 1 cup granulated sugar
- ½ tsp cinnamon (ground)

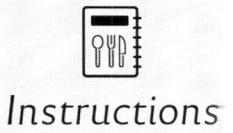
Instructions

1. You'll need a food processor or a blender for this first step. Toss your bran cereal, buttermilk, and flaxseed into the processor, mix the ingredients thoroughly and leave to settle for 30 minutes.
2. Preheat your oven to 350 °F.
3. While you wait for the oven to heat, you can start covering your muffin pan with cooking spray.
4. Going back to your mixture of ingredients, toss three bananas into the mix and blend once more until the batter is completely smooth.
5. Next, combine the nutmeg, salt, cinnamon, baking powder, and flour into a bowl and whisk.
6. Add this combination to the mixture in the food processor and pulse again until smooth.
7. Now for the fun part! Fill each muffin cup with batter, trying to get them as even as possible.
8. Once complete, slice the last banana into small, round discs and place one piece on each muffin.
9. Next, bake the muffins in the oven for 20-25 minutes (you will know they are ready when you stick a fork or toothpick inside and it comes out clean).
10. Once they are browned and ready, you can remove the muffins and leave them to cool down for a few moments before enjoying them.

MIXED BERRY AND BANANA SMOOTHIE

Cooking time: 10 minutes

Why We Love it

This recipe is quick to prepare and you can whip it up and take it with you when you need that extra kick to get through the day. The banana and yogurt will keep you feeling full throughout the day, and it tastes smooth, sweet, and refreshing Enjoy!

Nutrition facts

Servings: 2

Carbs: 70 g

Protein: 9 g

Fat: 5 g

Net carbs: 63 g

Calorie count per serving: 343

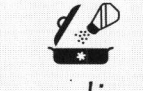

Ingredients

- 2 bananas
- ⅛ cup honey
- ⅓ cup Greek yogurt
- 1 cup milk
- 2 cups of frozen mixed berries

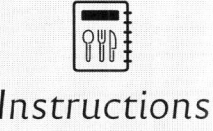

Instructions

1. Slice the banana into discs and simply toss all the above ingredients into a blender until the batch is smooth. If need be, you can add extra honey if you feel the smoothie isn't sweet enough.
2. Pour the smoothie into a glass and you can store any leftovers in the fridge for tomorrow.
3. Enjoy!

SUPERFOOD OATMEAL

Cooking time: 10 minutes

Why We Love it

Did you know that eating oatmeal can help boost the happy hormone serotonin in your brain? I'm not kidding! Oatmeal is one of the best foods you can eat to keep you energized, focused, and sustained for the rest of the day. This recipe also includes chia seeds which are packed with antioxidants and protein, as well as flaxseeds for omega and cinnamon for added flavor and zest.

Nutrition facts

Servings: 1

Carbs: 28 g

Protein: 5 g

Fat: 3 g

Net carbs: 24 g

Calorie count per serving: 160

Ingredients

- 1 tsp chia seeds
- ½ cup oats
- ¼ cup blueberries
- 1 tsp flax seeds (ground)
- ¼ tsp cinnamon
- 1 cup almond milk (unsweetened)

Instructions

1. Excluding the blueberries, mix together all the ingredients into a bowl.
2. You can then place the bowl in the microwave for two to three minutes, pausing to stir the mixture halfway through.
3. Once the oatmeal is cooked, you can simply sprinkle the top with blueberries, grab a spoon, and dig in!

ANTI-INFLAMMATORY SUPERFOOD TURMERIC BERRY SMOOTHIE

Cooking time: 2 minutes

Why We Love it

This recipe is not only easy to make but it's also exceptionally good for you! Turmeric is well-known for its high antioxidant count, anti-inflammatory properties, and pain relief. The remaining ingredients are also very high in vitamins, minerals, and antioxidants, making this the perfect addition to a healthy, balanced diet (Geimer, 2021). Plus, it will only take you a couple of minutes to prepare!

Nutrition facts

Servings: 2

Carbs: 30 g

Protein: 2 g

Fat: 1 g

Net carbs: 26 g

Calorie count per serving: 119

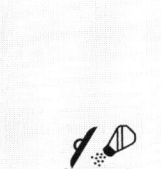
Ingredients

- 1 handful of kale or spinach (the choice is up to you)
- 1 banana
- coconut (shredded)
- hemp seeds
- granola
- fruit of choice
- 1 pinch chia seeds
- 1 ½ cup of mixed berries
- ½ cup of coconut or almond milk
- 2 tsp turmeric powder

Instructions

1. Simply toss all of the above ingredients into a blender (except for the chia and hemp seeds), and combine until the mixture is completely smooth.
2. Once blended, toss the seeds on top as well as any other toppings you desire and enjoy!

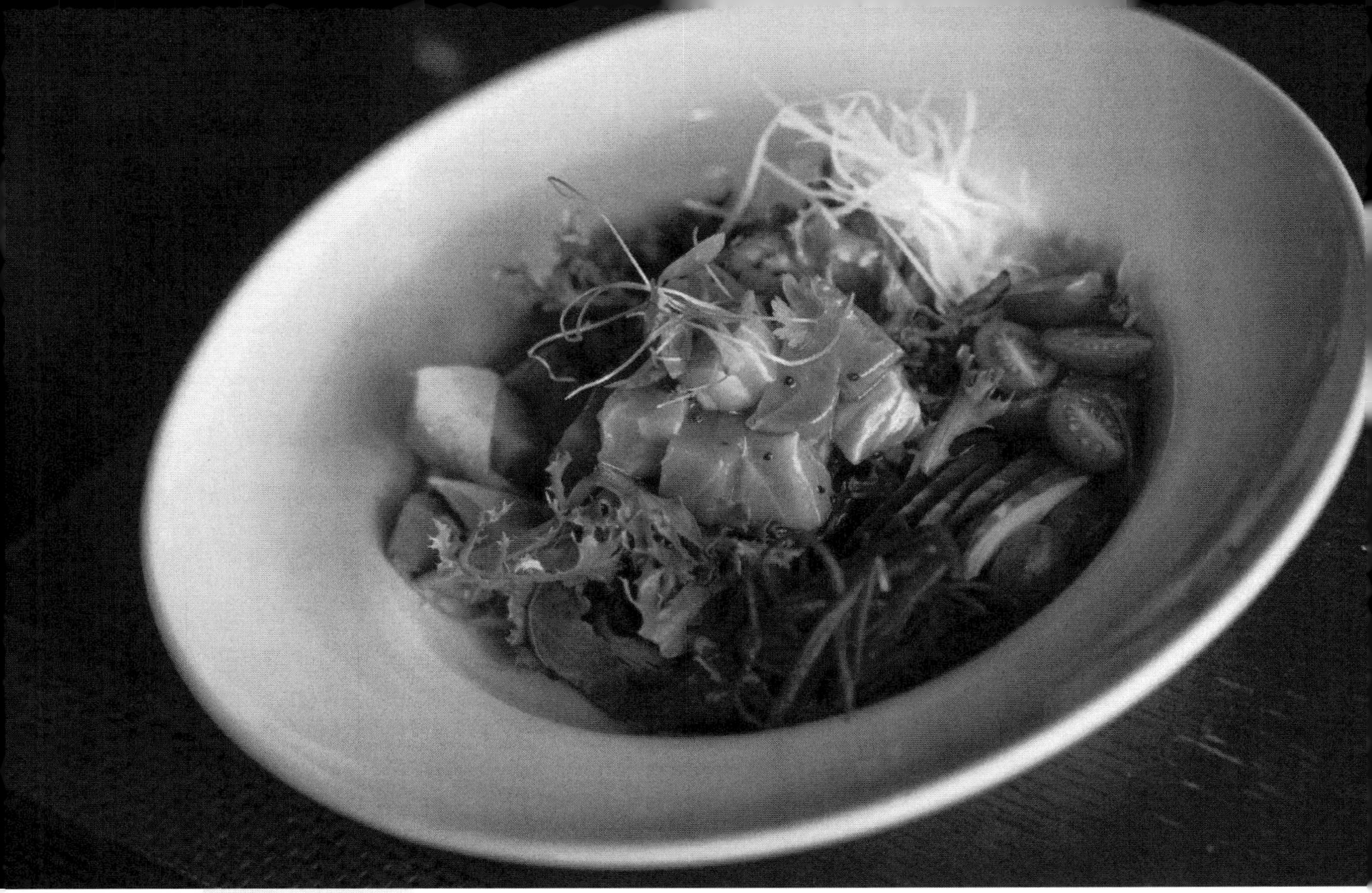

THAI SALMON AND CARROT SALAD

Cooking time: 30 minutes

Why We Love it

Salmon is jam-packed with omega 3's, vitamin D, B12, selenium, and various other important vitamins and minerals that help give you that youthful spring in your step. In fact, eating foods high in omega 3's is extremely important for older women as it helps to prevent osteoporosis and prevents inflammation associated with joint pain (Kingsley, 2021).

Nutrition facts

Servings: 3
Carbs: 21 g
Protein: 35g

Fat: 49 g
Net carbs: 17 g
Calorie count per serving: 654

Ingredients

For Salad:
- ¼ cup chopped raw cashews
- 3 cups carrots (shredded)
- 1 cup fresh cilantro
- ½ cup green onion (chopped)

For Salmon:
- 1 lb fresh salmon fillet
- 1 tsp Himalayan salt
- 1 tbsp lime juice
- ½ tsp ground pepper

For Dressing:
- ½ tsp Himalayan salt
- ¼ cup butter
- red pepper flakes to taste
- 3 tbsp lime juice
- 2 tbsp sesame seeds
- ½ cup olive oil

Instructions

1. Simply combine the cashews, carrots, cilantro, and onion into a serving bowl.
2. Next, pour some oil on the grill and set it on medium heat.
3. On the side of the fish without skin, rub the salt, lime juice, and pepper in for flavor.
4. Very gently place the fish with the skin facing upward on the grill and watch it carefully as you don't want to burn the meat.
5. Watch the fish until it develops a little bit of color and then flip it over so that the skin is facing downward. To tell whether your fish is ready, take note of the color. The inside should be slightly pinker than the outside, and you shouldn't have any problems slicing through.
6. To prepare the sauce, simply mix the salt, butter, red pepper flakes, lime juice, sesame seeds, and olive oil together in a salad dressing container and shake until thoroughly mixed.
7. Lastly, pour the dressing over your crisp, tasty carrot salad and mix it in.
8. Simply dish your salad onto a plate and toss your piece of salmon on top, pouring the dressing over the final product. Enjoy!

WARM KALE QUINOA SALAD

Cooking time: 15 minutes

As I have mentioned several times in this book, kale and quinoa are two incredibly healthy food choices. Put together, they create a dynamic duo! This salad is bursting with flavor and texture with fiber, minerals, and vitamins to keep you youthful, energized and glowing.

Why We Love it

Nutrition facts

Servings: 4

Carbs: 38 g

Protein: 13 g

Fat: 11 g

Net carbs: 32 g

Calorie count per serving: 377

Ingredients

- ¼ cup red onion (sliced in wedges)
- ⅛ tsp salt
- 2 cups of shredded chicken
- 1 sweet potato
- 1 ½ cups of chicken broth
- ¾ cup dry quinoa (rinsed and drained)
- 1 tsp dijon vinaigrette
- 1 apple quartered and sliced thinly
- 6 cups trimmed kale

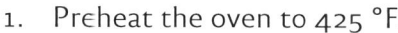

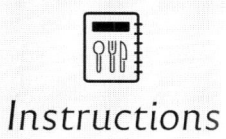
Instructions

1. Preheat the oven to 425 °F.
2. Peel your sweet potato and slice into wedges.
3. Take a baking tray, place the wedges into the pan, sprinkle with some salt, and drizzle with olive oil.
4. Place the tray in the oven to roast (uncovered) for 15-20 minutes.
5. While you wait for the potatoes, grab a large skillet and heat the quinoa and broth until they come to a boil, then turn down the heat.
6. Leave them to simmer for approximately 15 minutes (you'll know it's ready once there is no more water and the quinoa is soft).
7. Using the same skillet, heat one tbsp of olive oil on medium heat, then toss in the onion to cook for five minutes until browned.
8. Next, toss in the kale for an additional two to three minutes (make sure to turn them over frequently).
9. Grab a serving bowl; toss in the kale, as well as the chicken, sweet potato, apple slices, quinoa, and vinaigrette. Enjoy!

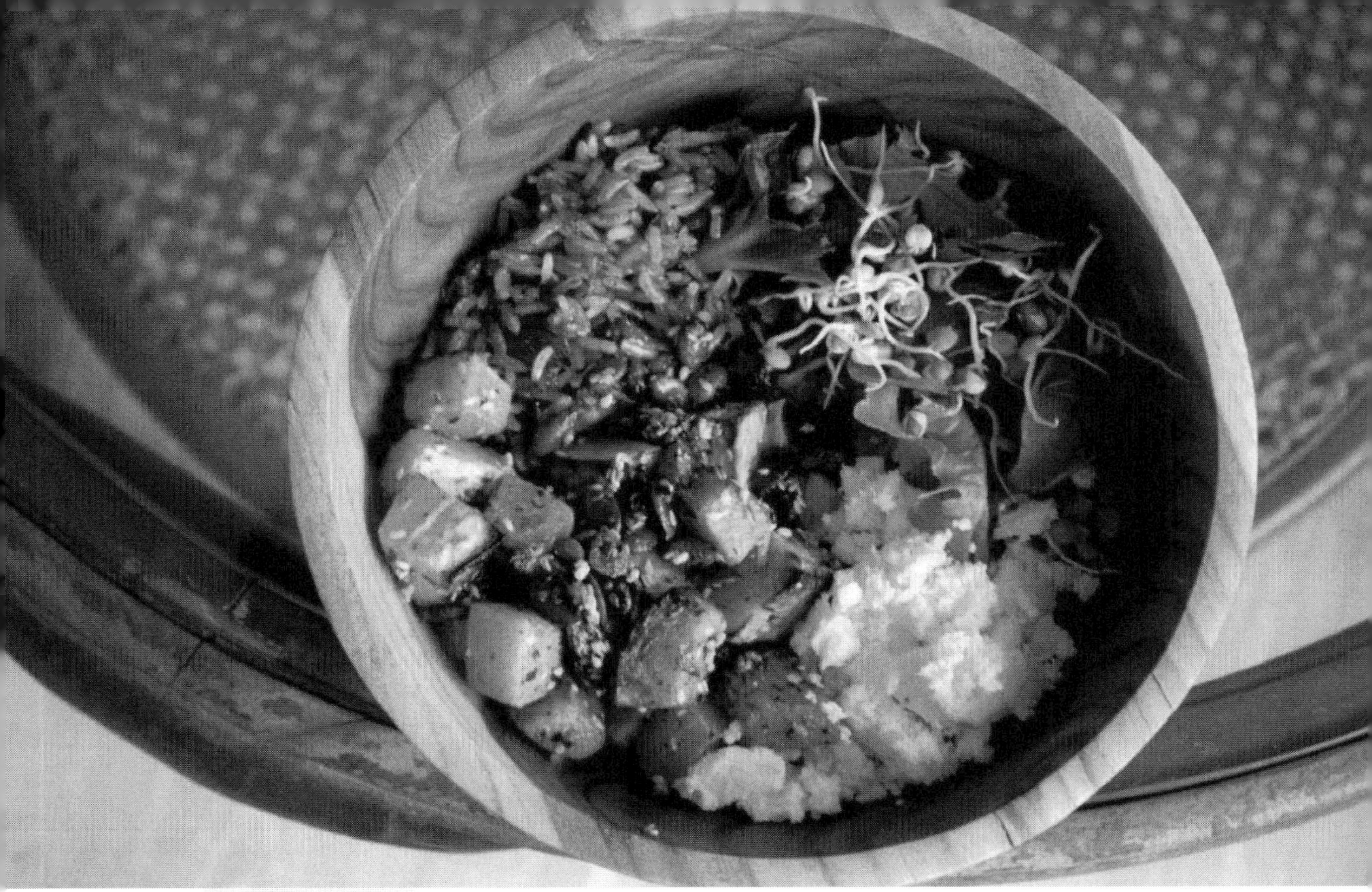

SWEET POTATO BUDDHA BOWL WITH CHICKPEAS

Cooking time: 45 minutes

Why We Love it

The Buddha bowl is a very special kind of dish and supposedly originated from the Buddhists making their rounds and filling their bowls with a variety of exotic, nutritious foods. This lovely dish will take you 30 minutes to prepare, and I can assure you that it will be well worth your time! This is a plant-based dish, but it still contains a rich, exotic flavor with all the protein, antioxidants, and minerals that you could ask for.

Nutrition facts

Servings: 1
Carbs: 62 g
Protein: 13.2 g
Fat: 21 g
Net carbs: 50.6 g
Calorie count per serving: 474

Ingredients

For Vegetables:
- salt and pepper to taste
- 12 large handfuls of kale
- 2 small sweet potatoes (halved)
- 1 bunch of broccolini
- ½ medium red onion (sliced in wedges)

For Tahini Sauce:
- ½ juiced lemon (medium)
- ¼ cup Tahini
- 1 tbsp maple syrup
- 2-4 tbsp hot water

For Chickpeas:
- ¼ tsp turmeric
- ¾ tsp garlic powder
- 1 tsp cumin
- ¾ tsp chilli powder
- 1 15 oz. can of chickpeas
- ½ tsp oregano

Instructions

1. Preheat the oven to 425 °F.
2. Grab a baking sheet and lay out the onions and sweet potatoes evenly, spreading them with oil and placing the potatoes skin down on the baking sheet.
3. After ten minutes of baking, you can remove the baking tray and add the broccolini, flipping the sweet potatoes as you do so.
4. Drizzle the broccoli with oil, salt, and pepper and bake for a further ten minutes.
5. Once the ten minutes are up you can toss in the kale, drizzled with salt, pepper, and oil, and place the tray back into the oven for an additional five minutes.
6. Grab a bowl and toss in your chickpeas while you heat up a medium-sized skillet
7. Throw in your seasoning over the chickpeas and wait for the skillet to heat up, then toss them into the pan (make sure that you grease the pan with one tbsp of oil first).
8. For the next ten minutes, wait for the chickpeas to cook while stirring occasionally, and make sure that they aren't browning too quickly (if they are, simply turn down the heat).
9. Next, you can start preparing the sauce by combining the tahini, lemon juice, and maple syrup.
10. Add some hot water if you need to add more liquid to the sauce, and combine the ingredients thoroughly then set them aside.
11. To serve, simply slice the sweet potatoes into smaller pieces and toss them in the bowl with the remaining ingredients; pour the sauce and chickpeas over the finished meal—Enjoy!

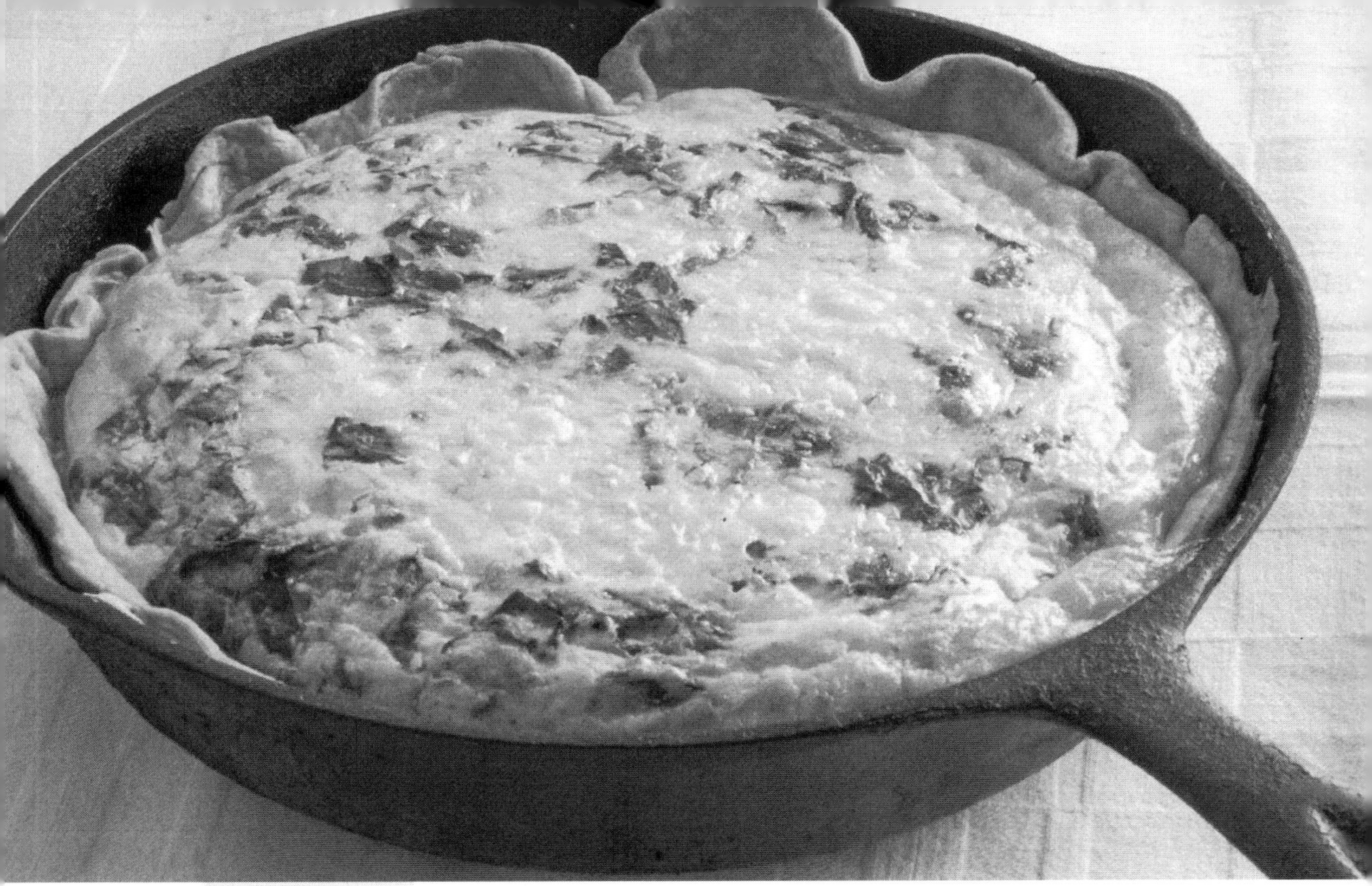

SPINACH QUICHE (WITHOUT THE CRUST)

Cooking time: 45 minutes

Why We Love it

This option is one of my personal favorites—it's packed with protein to keep you feeling fuller for longer, making it the perfect meal to enjoy before a fast to fuel up. In fact, one piece for breakfast will keep you going for hours! Plus, it contains a healthy dose of potassium which will help to prevent fasting-related headaches and balance the fluid in your system. Since you're preparing such a large portion, you can wrap and refrigerate leftovers as a convenient meal prep option for the rest of the week.

Nutrition facts

Servings: 8
Carbs: 7 g
Protein: 20 g
Fat: 13 g
Net carbs: 6 g
Calorie count per serving: 310

Ingredients

- 12 eggs
- 6 cups of fresh spinach
- ½ diced onion
- 1 pound of ground breakfast sausage
- 2 cups of diced mushrooms
- ½ cup of coconut milk (full-fat)
- 1 tsp salt
- 1 tsp pepper
- 1 tsp garlic powder
- 1 tsp Italian herbs
- butter, oil, or ghee (you can choose which works best)

Instructions

1. Preheat your oven to 400 °F.
2. While you wait for your oven to preheat you can start chopping up your onion and mushrooms.
3. For this next step, you'll need a cast iron pan or any other oven-friendly pan, which you will need to set on medium heat.
4. Toss in the sausage and onion and stir frequently.
5. After approximately 8 minutes your sausage should have fully browned and the onion would be translucent.
6. Once this happens, you can add in the mushrooms for another two minutes (they should soften completely).
7. While you wait, you can start chopping the spinach into smaller pieces.
8. Split all the eggs into a large bowl along with the coconut milk and whisk thoroughly.
9. Next, toss the spinach and coconut mixture into the bowl.
10. Revert back to your mixture of sausage, mushrooms, and onion and add this into the bowl; mix everything together thoroughly.
11. Make sure that your cast iron pan is thoroughly greased with butter, oil, or ghee, and place the mixture in the pan.
12. Bake for 30 minutes in the oven and make sure the egg is set.
13. You'll know the quiche is ready when the egg is no longer runny and the top is crispy and brown in color.
14. Finally, you can cut your quiche into 8-10 pieces and enjoy!

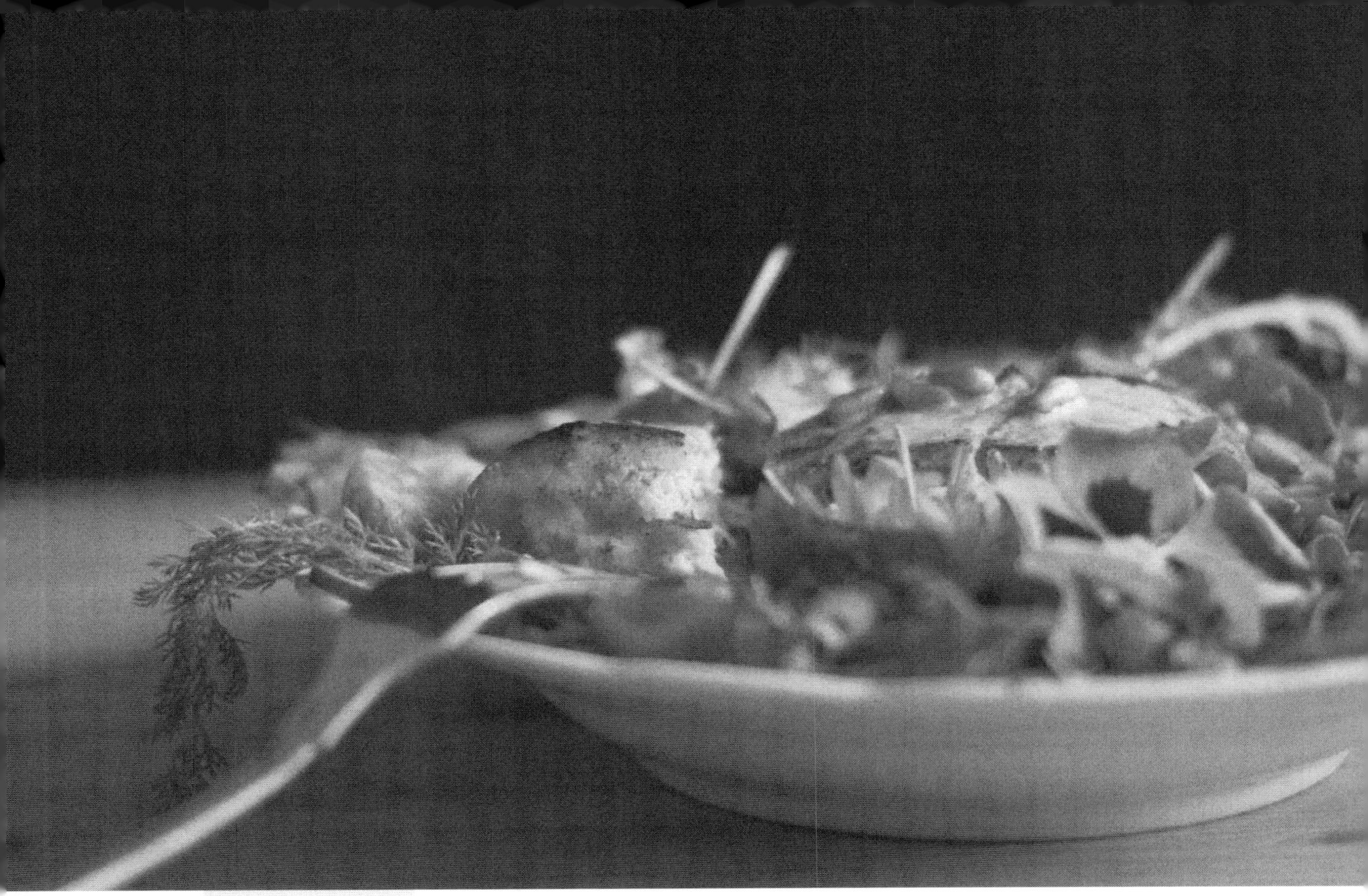

LEMON CHICKEN
AVOCADO SALAD

Cooking time: 30 minutes

Why We Love it

This next recipe is jam-packed with goodness! It contains plenty of healthy fats, protein, and fiber, and is perfect for a post-workout meal to maintain and build muscle while you progress through your fasting journey. It's also loaded with vitamins and antioxidants due to the added berries and kale. What more could you ask for in a meal?

Nutrition facts

Servings: 4
Carbs: 25 g
Protein: 8 g
Fat: 32 g
Net carbs: 19 g
Calorie count per serving: 254

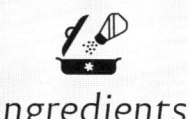

Ingredients

- 2 chicken breasts (skinless)
- 1 large portion of kale (stemless)
- ½ tbsp lemon zest
- 1 sprig rosemary
- 2 tsp Italian seasoning
- 1 cup of wheat berries (cooked)
- ½ cup pomegranate arils
- 2 tbsp olive oil
- 1 tsp dijon mustard
- 2 tsp minced garlic
- 1 ripe avocado
- 2 tbsp extra virgin olive oil
- 1 tsp peppercorns (pink)
- sea salt and black pepper to taste
- ½ cup roasted pine nuts
- 1 tsp honey
- ½ tsp grated lemon zest
- pea shoots (optional for garnish)

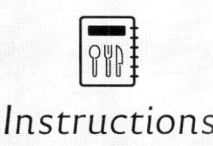

Instructions

1. Start by thoroughly cleaning the chicken breasts and placing them aside to drain.
2. Next, score the chicken pieces so that the marinade can seep in properly.
3. For your marinade, place the olive oil, honey, lemon zest, Italian seasoning, and minced garlic into a bowl and thoroughly combine with a pinch of salt and pepper.
4. Next, combine this marinade with the chicken and leave to fully marinate for approximately 15 minutes.
5. Preheat the oven to 375 °F.
6. Set a cast-iron skillet on the stove and turn the heat up to medium.
7. Toss in your marinated chicken breasts and cook until they are browned on both sides.
8. Next, transfer the skillet into the oven for approximately 10 minutes.
9. Take the kale and move it into your chosen serving dish and throw in your sliced avocado.
10. Once the chicken breasts are ready, slice them into small pieces and toss them into the salad.
11. Now, sprinkle your berries, nuts, peppercorns, and pomegranates evenly across the salad.
12. Garnish with the pea shoots if you wish.

CREAMY KABOCHA SQUASH AND ROASTED RED PEPPER PASTA

Cooking time: 30 minutes

Not only is this dish super tasty, but it's good for you too! You won't be able to tell the difference between regular pasta and this dish, except for the fact that this tastes better.

Why We Love it

Servings: 4

Carbs: 93.4 g

Protein: 17.8 g

Fat: 5.9 g

Net carbs: 0 g

Calorie count per serving: 501

Nutrition facts

Ingredients

- 1 head of garlic
- ½ medium onion (chopped)
- salt and pepper to taste
- 1 kabocha squash (small)
- ½ cup raw cashews
- 2-3 cups of vegetable broth
- 2 tbsp nutritional yeast
- 1 stalk chopped celery
- 1 medium chopped carrot
- ⅓ cauliflower florets

- ¾ cup basil
- 2 lbs gluten-free spaghetti noodles
- parmesan cheese
- ¼ red peppers (roasted)

Instructions

1. Grab a small pot of water and boil it, removing the pot once boiled and tossing the cashews in to soak for one hour (alternatively, you can leave them to soak in cool water overnight if you have the time).
2. Preheat the oven to 400°F and place your cooking rack in the middle of the oven.
3. Using a silicone mat or parchment paper, line your baking tray.
4. Next, wash and dry the kabocha squash and place it in the tray whole, leaving it to cook for 18-20 minutes.
5. Once the time is up, remove the squash from the oven and allow the squash to cool.
6. Vertically, slice the squash in half and remove the seeds and fiber with a spoon.
7. Slice the squash into one-inch wedges, trying to keep the wedges as even as possible.
8. Place seven slices of the squash onto the baking sheet (you can leave the rest for another time).
9. Remove any excess skin from the garlic by hand, taking a sharp knife and removing the head of the garlic so you can see the surface of the cloves.
10. Place the garlic down on the cut side alongside the florets, celery, carrots, and onions.
11. Drizzle some salt and pepper and place back into the oven for 40 minutes, making sure to flip after approximately 20 minutes.
12. With only 10 minutes to go before the vegetables are done, be sure to start on the pasta.
13. Once you have removed the baking sheet, leave the vegetables out to cool and remove the skin from the kabocha and toss the pieces into a blender (you can toss the skin if you wish).
14. Toss the soaked cashews into the blender along with the garlic cloves, vegetables, red peppers, yeast, vegetable broth, salt, and pepper.
15. Blend thoroughly until smooth, and feel free to add in one more cup of vegetable broth if required.
16. Toss in the basil, but be sure to pulse it as blending it may turn the sauce a strange color.
17. Now you are ready to eat! Sprinkle some fresh parmesan and pepper and enjoy!

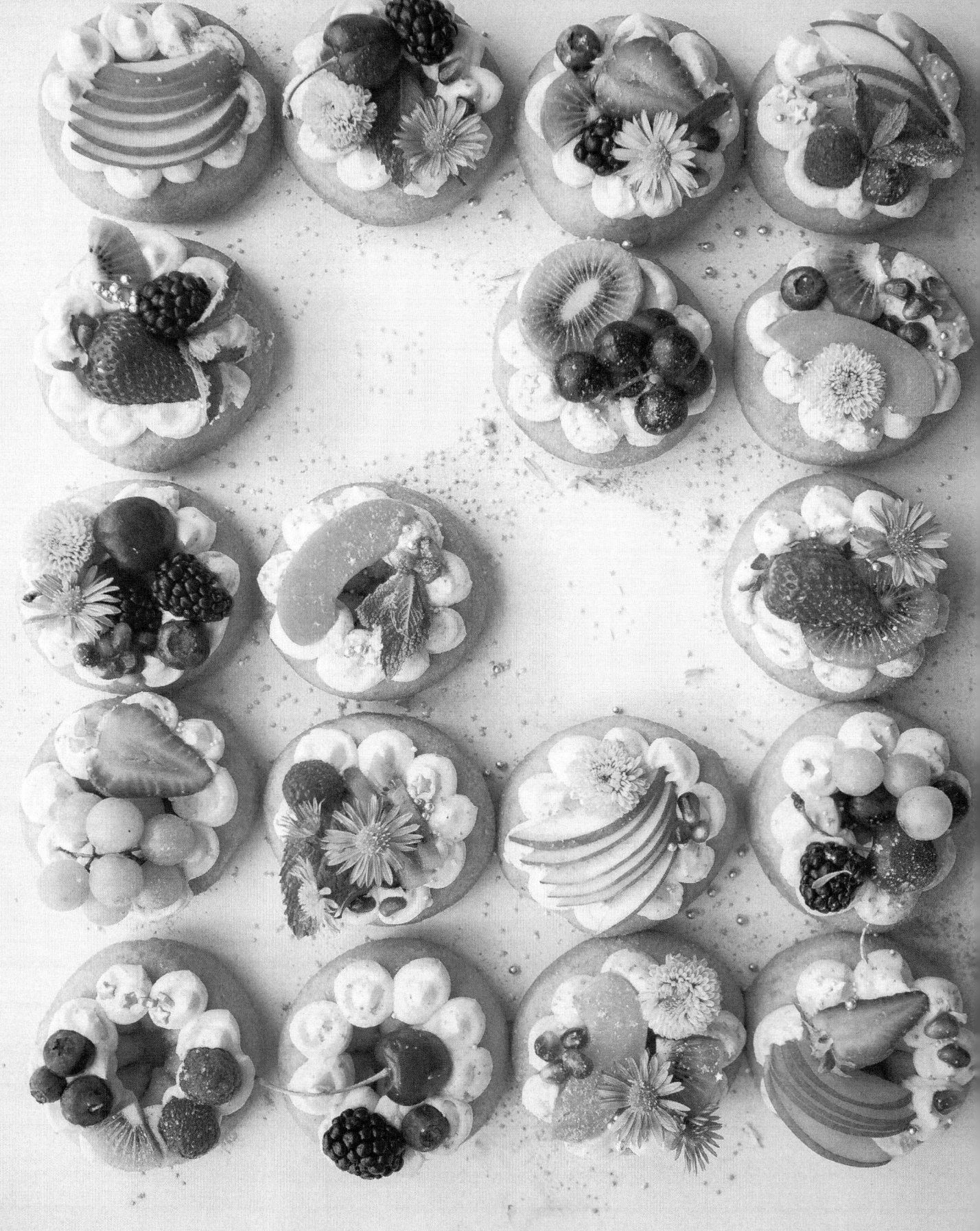

DELICIOUS MEALS UNDER 500 CALORIES FOR FASTING DAYS

This section will focus on some tasty meals under 500 calories that you can prepare for your fasting days. Not only are they low-calorie, but they're full of vitamins and minerals to keep you energized and feeling great!

SLOW-COOKED SEAFOOD RAMEN

Cooking time: 2-3 hours

This delicious treat is packed with protein, antioxidants, and a rich, flavorful taste. It doesn't take a lot of effort to prepare and it packs all the benefits with the fewest calories (only 307 calories per serving), making it the perfect anti-aging and weight loss choice!

Why We Love it

Nutrition facts

Servings: 4

Carbs: 39 g

Protein: 29.5 g

Fat: 2.7 g

Net carbs: 37 g

Calorie count per serving: 307

Ingredients

- 64 oz. bone broth
- 4.6 oz ramen
- ¼ cup chopped kale
- 1 lb mixed seafood
- 2 minced garlic cloves
- 1 tsp sesame oil
- 1 tsp salt
- 2 sliced green onions
- ¼ tsp pepper
- 2 tbsp reduced-sodium soy sauce
- 2 tbsp rice vinegar
- ½ lb sliced tomatoes

Instructions

1. Excluding the seafood, ramen, and kale, toss all of the ingredients into a slow cooker.
2. Cook on high heat for 2-3 hours, or alternatively, on a low heat for 4-6 hours.
3. Toss in the kale, ramen, and seafood for an extra 15-30 minutes.
4. Enjoy!

GINGER MAPLE
GLAZED SALMON
Cooking time: 30 minutes

Why We Love it

This super healthy meal is perfect for a fasting day lunch, with protein, healthy fats, and omega 3's. The best aspect of this meal is the fact that it only takes 10 minutes to prepare, and it's full of vitamins and potassium, making it the perfect addition to any fasting guide (Mazzoni, 2021).

Nutrition facts

Servings: 1
Carbs: 16 g
Protein: 16 g
Fat: 4 g
Net carbs: 14 g
Calorie count per serving: 155

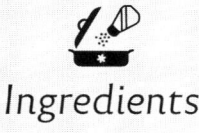
Ingredients

- 1 clove garlic
- 2-4 oz. wild salmon fillet
- 1 tsp maple syrup
- 2 tsp sesame oil
- 1 slice fresh ginger
- 1 tsp soy sauce

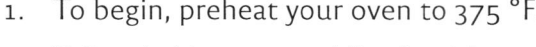

Instructions

1. To begin, preheat your oven to 375 °F.
2. Take a baking tray and line it with parchment paper.
3. While you wait for the oven, chop the ginger and garlic.
4. Taking a small bowl, mix all the ingredients together to create your sauce (excluding the salmon).
5. Take the salmon and place it into the baking tray.
6. Grab a teaspoon and pour the sauce evenly over the salmon.
7. Place the salmon on the middle grid in the oven and cook for 15-20 minutes until it turns a light golden color.

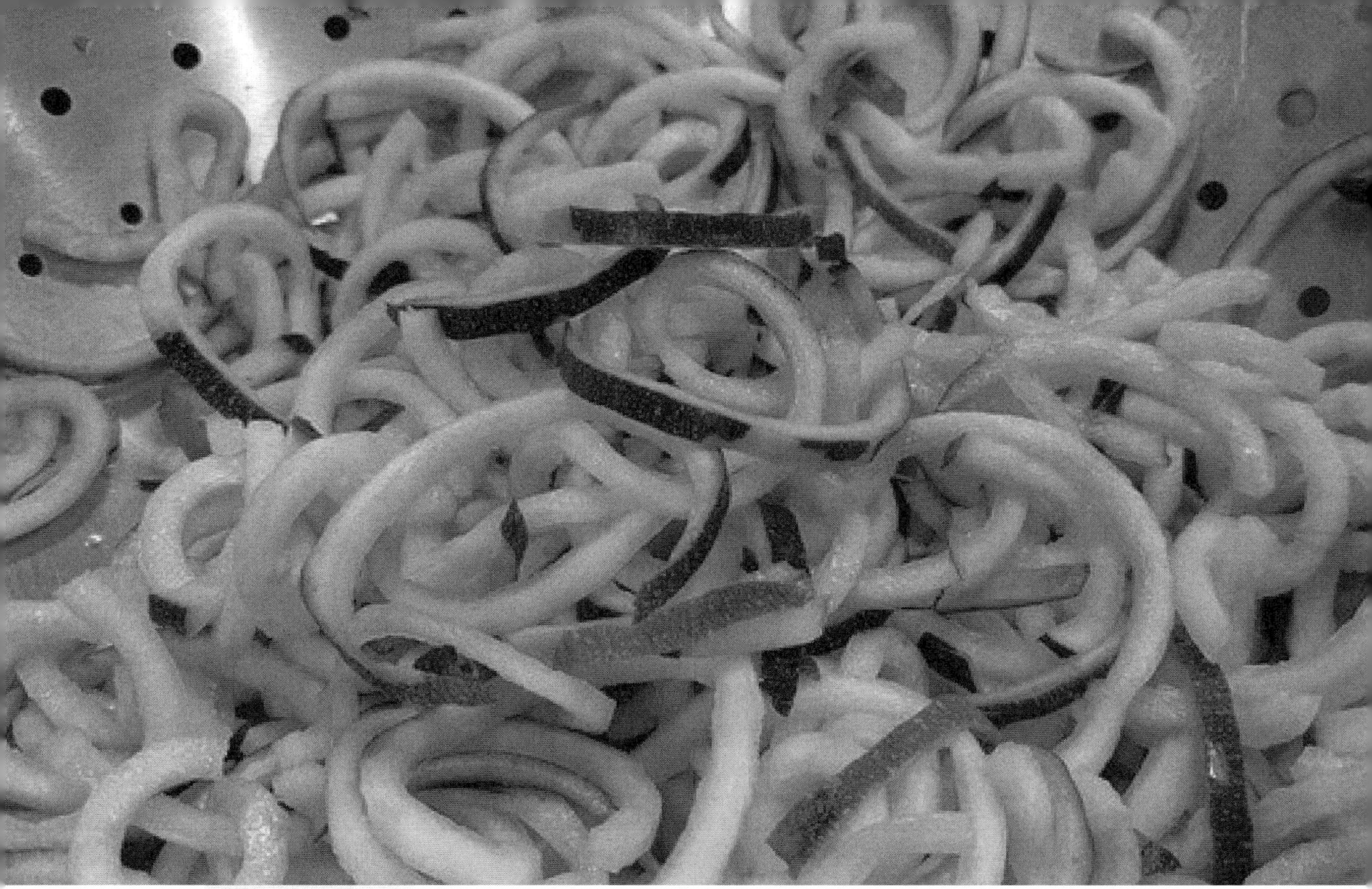

CAPRESE ZOODLES

Cooking time: 35 minutes

Why We Love it

If you're looking to cut your calories and carbs and still enjoy a tasty, wholesome meal, then this recipe is perfect for any lunch or dinner option.

Nutrition facts

Servings: 4
Carbs: 14 g
Protein: 16 g
Fat 17 g
Net carbs: 11 g
Calorie count per serving: 272

Ingredients

- 4 zucchinis (large)
- 2 tbsp extra virgin olive oil
- 2 cups of cherry tomatoes
- 2 tbsp balsamic vinegar
- black pepper to taste
- 1 cup mozzarella balls
- ¼ fresh basil leaves
- pinch of kosher salt

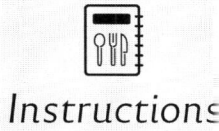

Instructions

1. For this first step, you'll need a spiralizer on hand! You will need to take your zucchini and place them in the spiralizer to make zoodles.
2. Grab a large bowl and toss the zoodles, salt, pepper, and olive oil inside, allowing them to sit for 15 minutes
3. Once the 15 minutes are up, toss in the tomatoes, mozzarella, and basil
4. Lastly, drizzle some balsamic vinegar on the top and dig in!

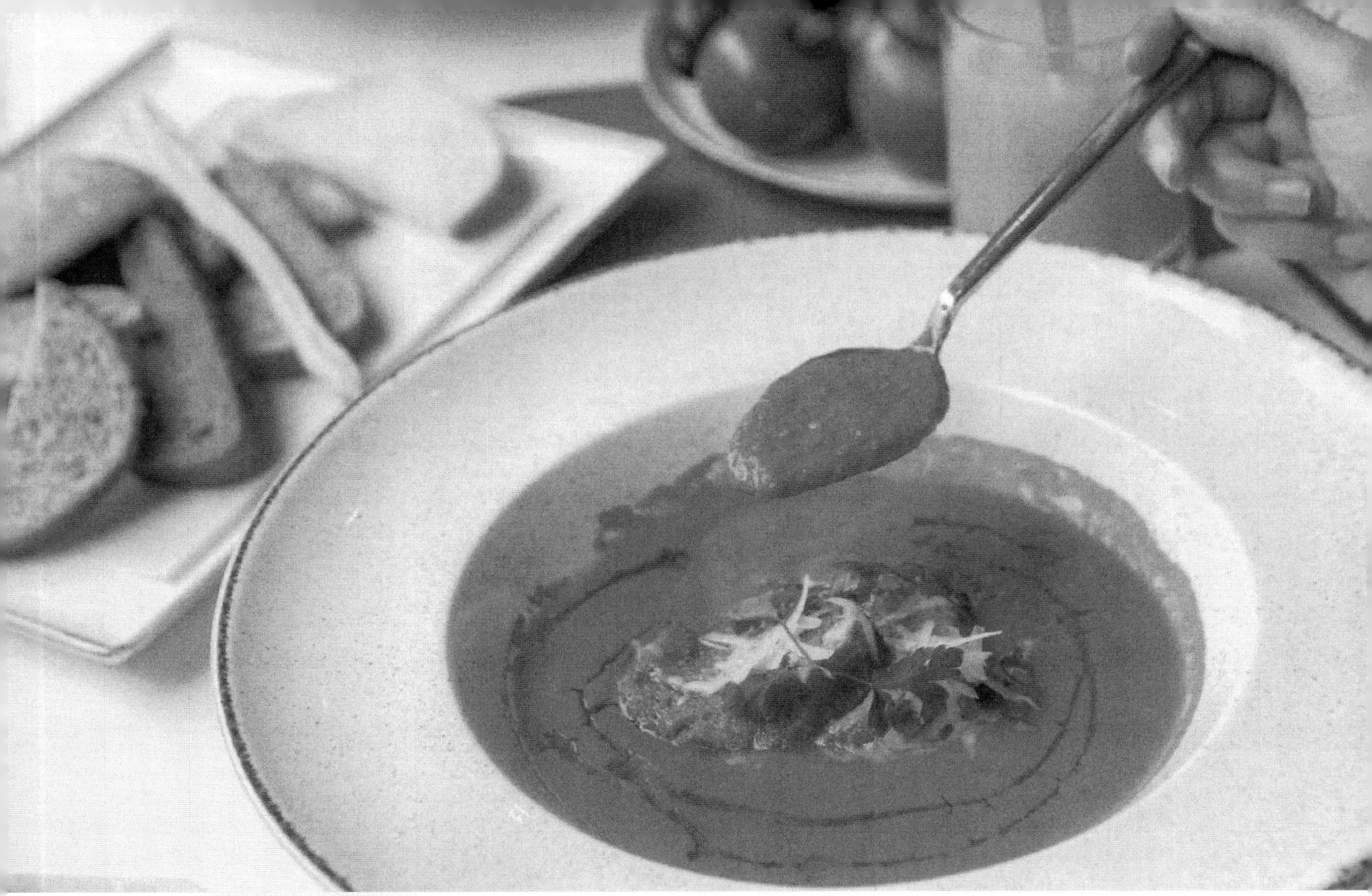

MEATBALL AND TOMATO SOUP

Cooking time: 20 minutes

Why We Love it

This soup is perfect for a lunchtime meal and will keep you feeling fuller for longer. Its rich and tasty flavor will satisfy your taste buds and the added spinach, garlic, and meatballs will provide you with the nutrients your body craves.

Nutrition facts

Servings: 4
Carbs: 6.1 g
Protein: 17 g
Fat: 12 g
Net carbs: 5.4 g
Calorie count per serving: 183

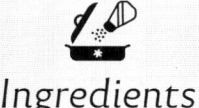
Ingredients

- 2 cans of tomatoes (chopped)
- 2 sliced red peppers
- 12 pork meatballs
- 3.5 oz. couscous
- ¼ tsp chili flakes
- 1 finely chopped onion
- 5.3 oz baby spinach
- ½ handful of dried basil
- 1 crushed garlic clove
- 2 cups of vegetable stock
- grated parmesan to taste

Instructions

1. Grab a saucepan and begin to heat up the oil, then fry the onions and peppers for approximately seven minutes.
2. Once the seven minutes are up, you can toss in the chili flakes and garlic and stir for an additional one minute.
3. Add in the vegetable stock, tomatoes, and couscous and bring them to a simmer
4. Next, season the soup to give it flavor and toss in the meatballs and the baby spinach.
5. Allow the soup to simmer for approximately seven minutes.
6. Once the time is up, you can ladle the soup into bowls and sprinkle with parmesan and basil.
7. Enjoy!

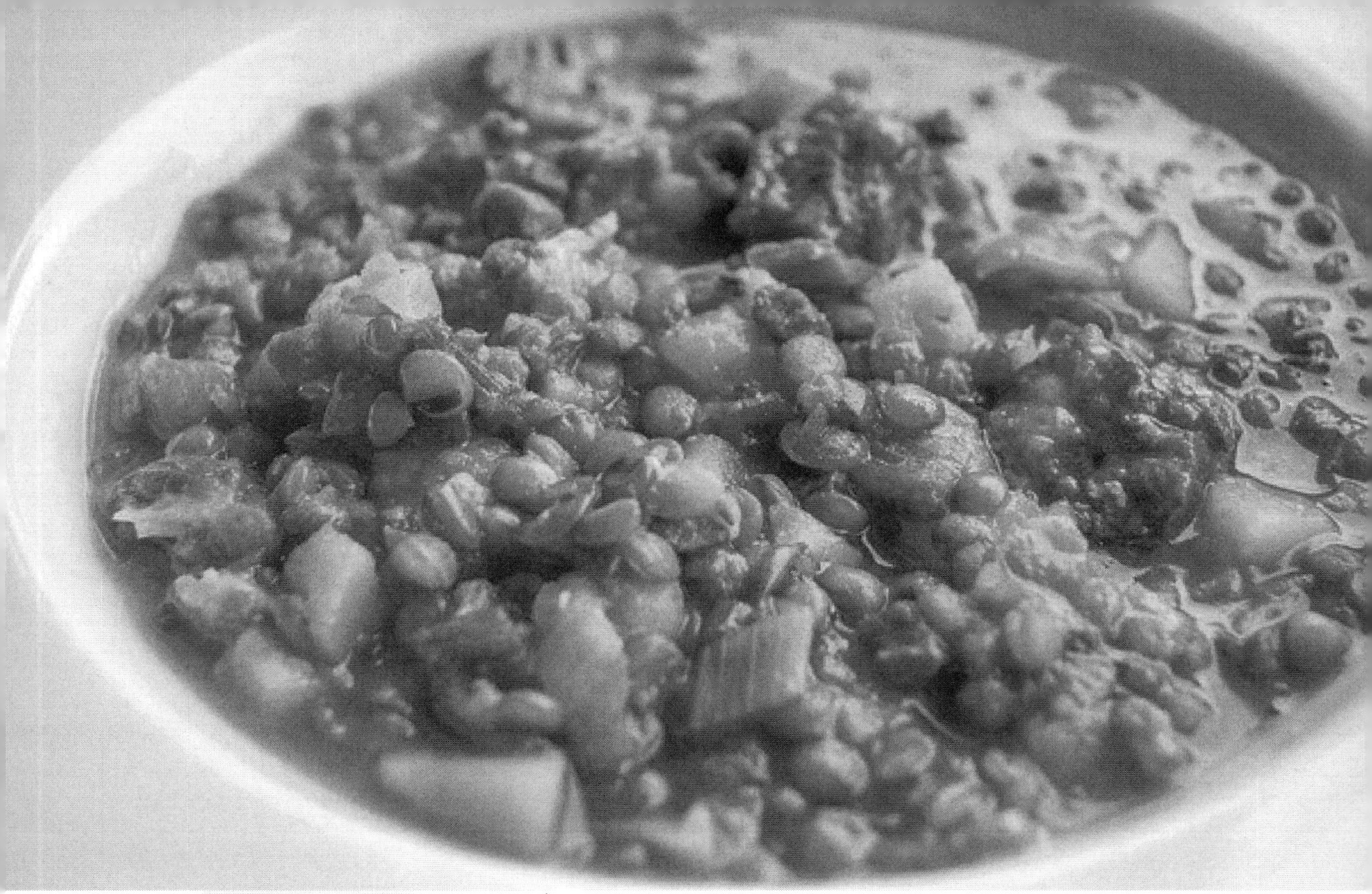

LENTIL SOUP

Cooking time: 20 minutes

Why We Love it

When it comes to fasting, I'm all about soup! Not only is it filling, but it's also full of nutrients. This particular soup recipe contains one of my favorite fasting foods—lentils! You can prepare this soup, freeze it, and save it for a later date to enjoy.

Nutrition facts

Servings: 4

Carbs: 20 g

Protein: 17 g

Fat: 12 g

Net carbs: 14.5 g

Calorie count per serving: 139

Ingredients

- 1 ½ cups of brown or green lentils
- 1 cup of water
- 1 tbsp paprika
- 1 garlic clove
- 1 tsp kosher salt
- 1 tbsp oregano (dried)
- 2 large carrots
- 3 cups of baby spinach
- 1 bulb of fennel
- 1 medium yellow onion
- ¼ cup olive oil
- 1-quart vegetable broth
- 28 ounces of fire-roasted tomatoes

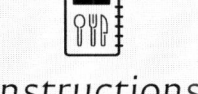

Instructions

1. Start by grabbing a chopping board and dicing the onion and the fennel.
2. Next, peel and slice the carrots.
3. Grate the garlic and set it aside with the rest of your ingredients.
4. Set the heat to medium and grab a large pot to heat up the olive oil.
5. Next, toss in the fennel and onion and allow them to cook for approximately seven minutes.
6. Once done, you can add in the lentils, broth, carrots, tomatoes, paprika, salt, water, and dried oregano.
7. Bring all the above ingredients to a simmer for approximately 25 minutes (you'll know it's ready when the lentils are soft).
8. Lastly, toss in the garlic and spinach, making sure that you stir the ingredients thoroughly.
9. After five minutes you can dish up your delicious meal and enjoy!

LEMON GARLIC BUTTER CHICKEN WITH GREEN BEANS SKILLET

Cooking time: 30 minutes

This next recipe is another one of my favorites due to its incredibly delicious flavor! This is the perfect pre-fast meal to enjoy for lunch or dinner that will satisfy your taste buds and keep you feeling full.

Why We Love it

Nutrition facts

Servings: 3
Carbs: 17 g
Protein: 36 g
Fat: 45 g
Net carbs: 10 g
Calorie count per serving: 616

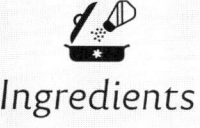
Ingredients

- 16 oz. green beans (frozen)
- 3-6 deboned chicken thighs (skinless)
- 4 minced garlic cloves
- 3 tbsp butter (a healthier option is ghee)
- 1 tbsp Sriracha hot sauce
- ½ cup chopped parsley
- 1 tsp onion powder
- ½ cup chicken stock
- 1 tsp paprika
- ¼ teaspoon crushed chili flakes
- ½ lemon for flavor and garnish (optional)
- salt and pepper to taste

Instructions

1. Grab a small bowl and mix together the paprika, onion powder, salt, and pepper.
2. Next, generously season the chicken thighs and place them aside.
3. For the green beans, you'll need to place them in a microwave-friendly bowl with ½ cup of water.
4. Cook the beans in the microwave for approximately four to five minutes until they are slightly crisp.
5. Next, melt two tbsp of butter or ghee in a skillet and set the heat to medium.
6. Once the skillet has heated you can transfer the chicken thighs into the skillet and leave them to cook for approximately five to six minutes.
7. Flip the chicken and cook for a further five to six minutes. If you notice that the chicken is turning brown too quickly, turn the heat down slightly (use your discretion).
8. Once the chicken is fully cooked you can flip it onto a plate and set it aside.
9. Using the same skillet, turn the heat down and melt the rest of the butter (1 tbsp).
10. Toss in the chili flakes, parsley, garlic, beans, and hot sauce and allow them to cook for five minutes (stir often).
11. Add in the stock and lemon juice, reducing the sauce for a few minutes (it should gradually become thicker).
12. Toss the chicken thighs back into the pan and reheat slightly.
13. You can now transfer the chicken thighs onto a plate and season with more pepper, chili pepper, and parsley—Enjoy!

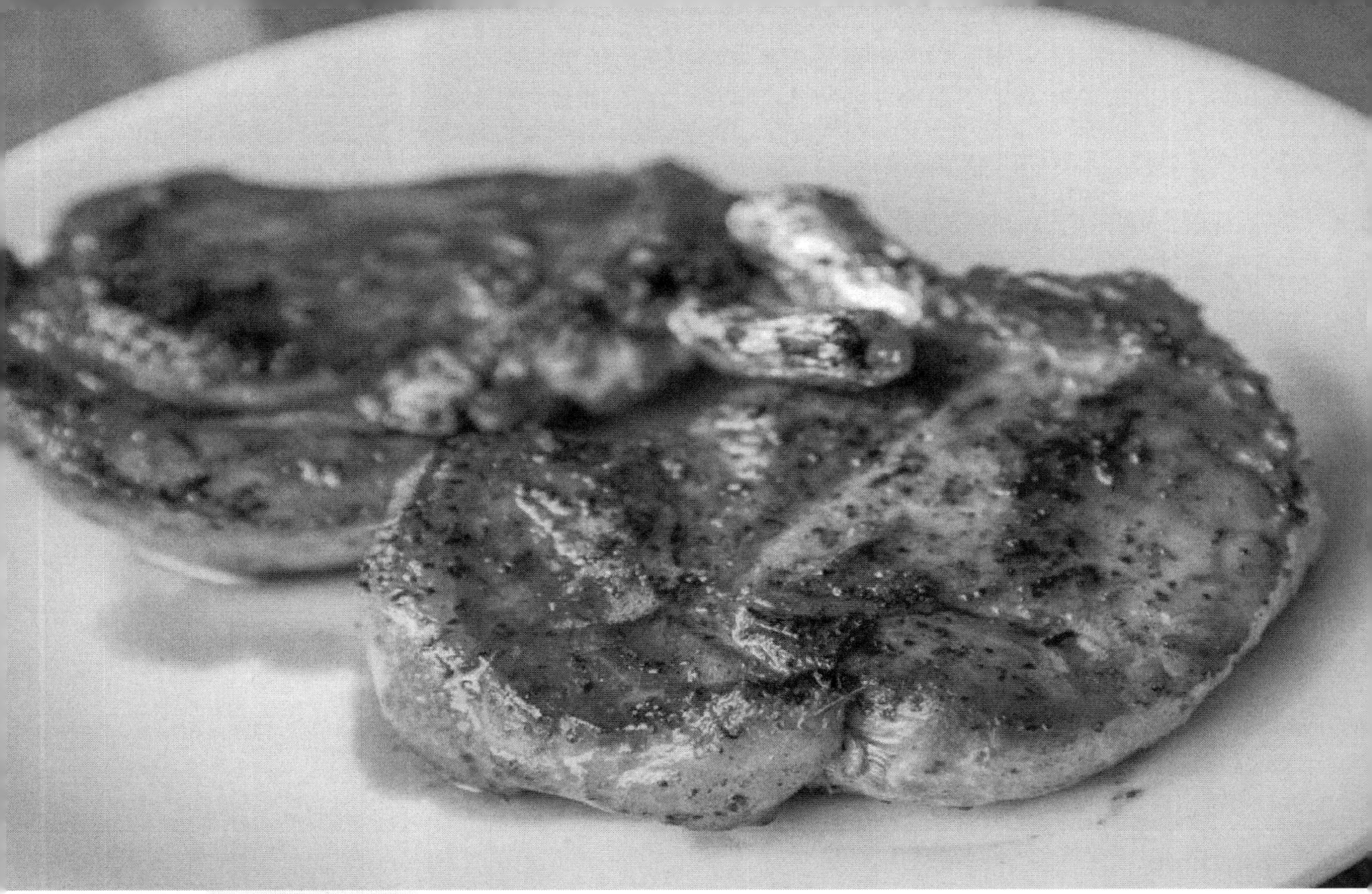

HONEY MUSTARD
PORK CHOPS

Cooking time: 35 minutes

Why We Love it

These honey-mustard pork chops with potato taste absolutely incredible and you'll be addicted once you try them! Be prepared for a melt-in-your-mouth experience with this recipe, bursting with flavor and character.

Nutrition facts

Servings: 4
Carbs: 27 g
Protein: 42 g
Fat: 27 g
Net carbs: 24 g
Calorie count per serving: 430

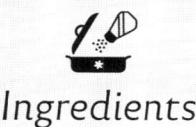

Ingredients

- 4 pork chops
- 1 tsp paprika (smoked)
- ⅓ cup mustard (whole grain)
- 1 tbsp lemon juice
- 1 lb baby yellow potatoes, rinsed and sliced into quarters
- One small handful of fresh parsley for garnish (chopped)
- salt and pepper to taste
- ¼ cup honey

Instructions

1. Grab a pot and boil some hot water, then toss in the quartered potatoes to boil for approximately eight minutes.
2. Once the potatoes have boiled you can remove them and drain them.
3. While you wait for the potatoes to drain, go ahead and season the pork chops on both sides, making sure to pat them dry before you do so.
4. Grab a large skillet and heat one tablespoon of butter and oil (one of each).
5. Once melted, toss the potatoes until they turn a golden hue; sautée every so often.
6. Once the potatoes are crisp and ready, you can transfer them to a plate.
7. Using the same skillet, add the pork chops in and cook for approximately three to four minutes, making sure that you flip them occasionally so both sides are evenly cooked.
8. Once the chops are cooked you can set them aside on another plate and pour the honey mustard back into the same skillet, making sure that you turn the heat down so it doesn't burn.
9. Allow the sauce to reduce for a moment and then toss the cooked potatoes back into the skillet (make sure they are thoroughly coated).
10. Once done, transfer the potatoes back onto a plate and return the pork chops back into the skillet to absorb the flavor of the honey mustard for about 30 seconds, then remove them.
11. Once the pork chops are fully coated you can remove them from the skillet and serve them up with your delicious, golden potatoes—enjoy!

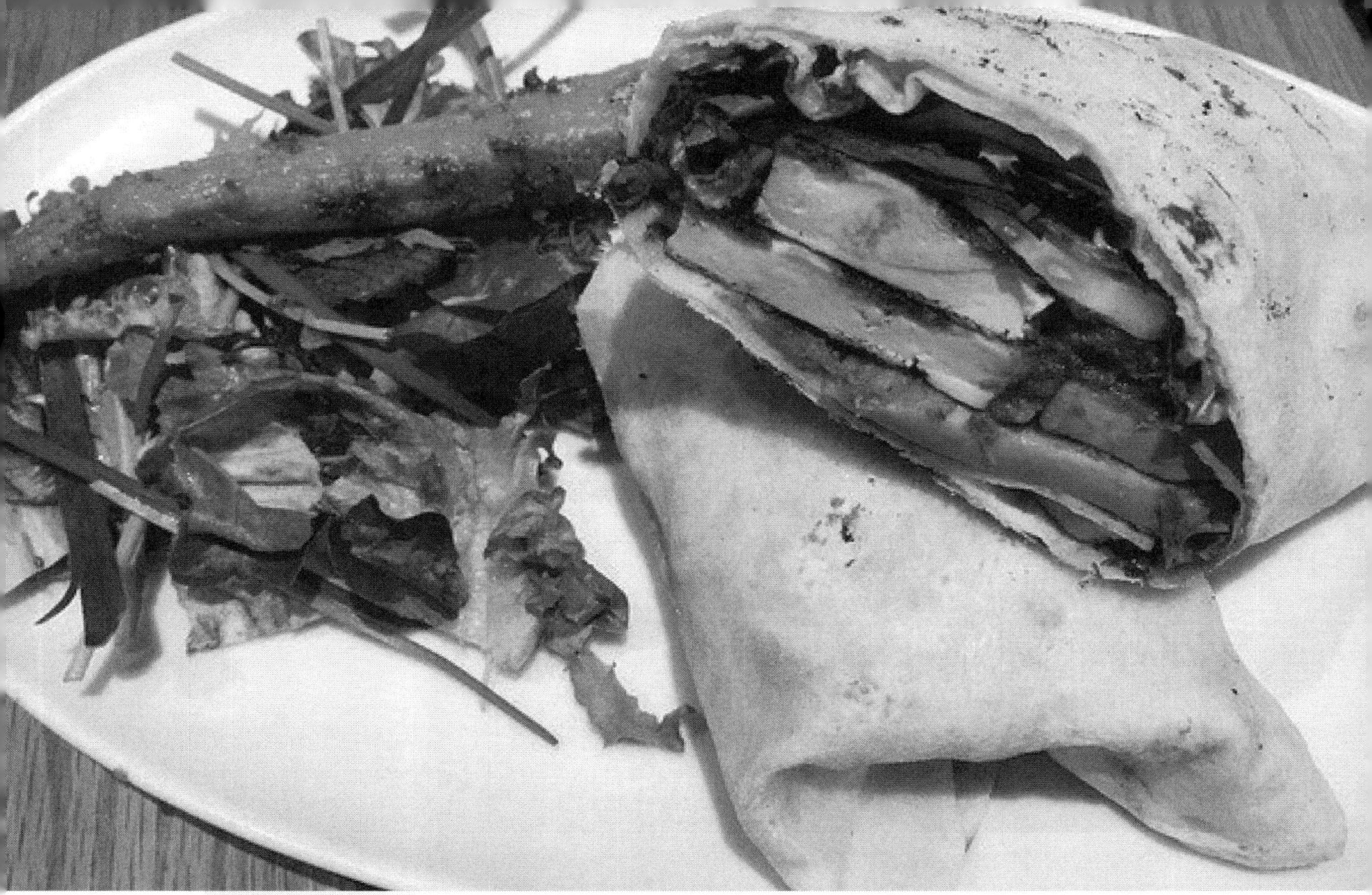

SPICY CHICKEN AND AVOCADO WRAP

Cooking time: 15 minutes

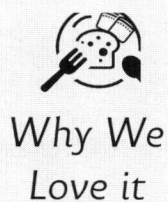

Why We Love it

This is the perfect lunch to whip up in preparation for breaking your fast and contains lean protein, healthy fats, and complex carbs. Essentially, you've hit the trifecta! In only 15 minutes you can whip up this tasty dish, so here's what to do.

Nutrition facts

Cooking time: 15 minutes

Servings: 2

Carbs: 32 g

Protein: 29 g

Fat: 16 g

Net carbs: 27 g

Calorie count per serving: 403

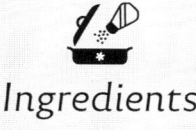
Ingredients

- 1 sliced chicken breast
- 1 halved avocado
- 1 tsp olive oil
- 1 chopped garlic clove
- 2 whole-wheat wraps
- ½ tsp chili powder (mild)
- 1 roasted red pepper
- 1 squeeze of lime juice
- 2 sprigs of coriander

Instructions

1. Start by combining the garlic, chili powder, and lime together with the chicken in a bowl.
2. Next, find a nonstick pan and quickly fry the chicken for a few minutes (be sure not to overcook it or it will be tough).
3. While you wait for the chicken, warm the wraps in the microwave. Try not to let the wraps dry out or they won't fold properly.
4. Grab your avocados and use a knife to spread them into the wraps, then add the peppers into the pan to warm them.
5. Add the chicken into the wrap with the warm peppers and sprinkle some coriander, then roll up the wrap, cut, and enjoy!

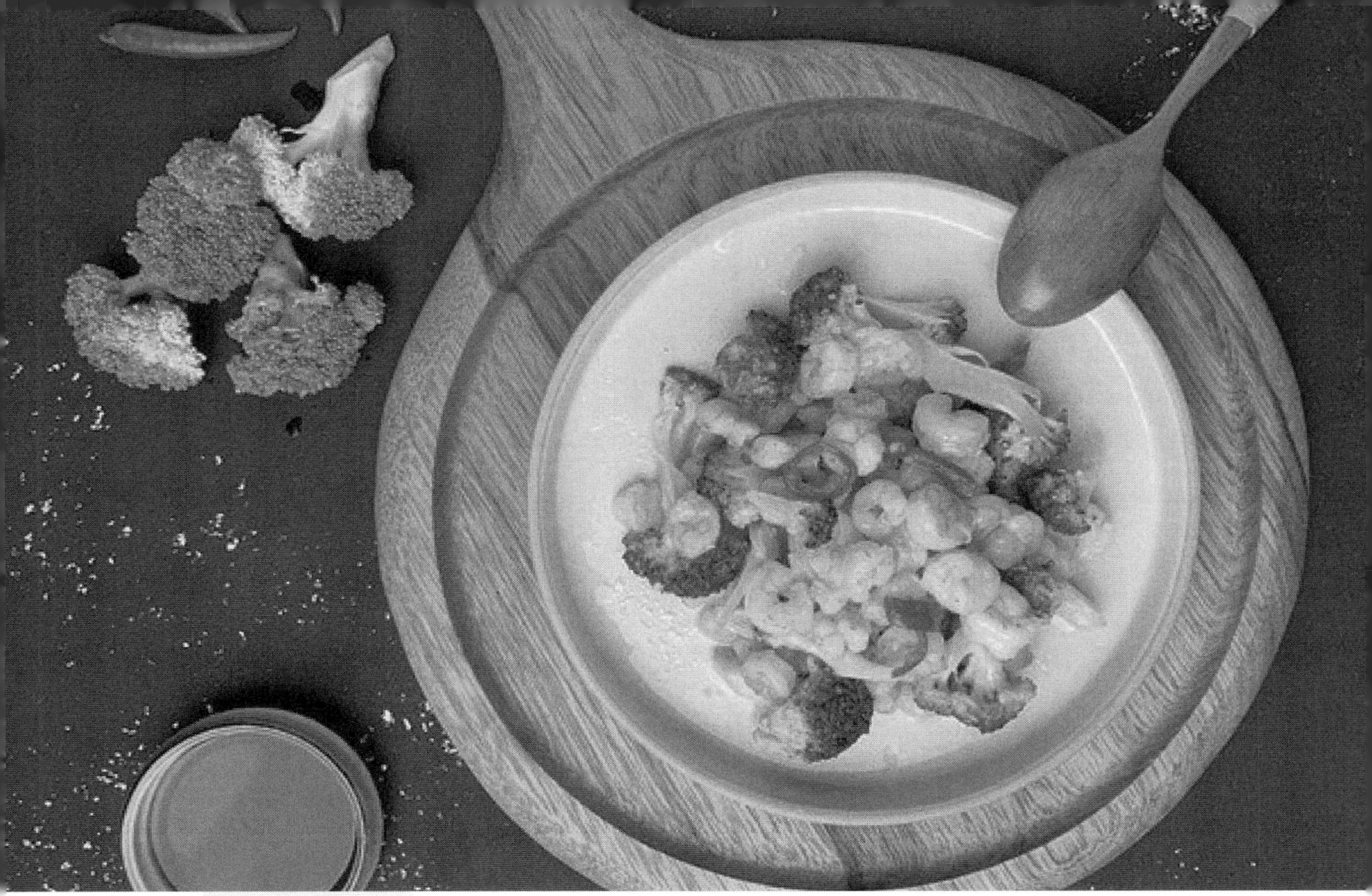

SHRIMP AND BROCCOLI

Cooking time: 20 minutes4

Why We Love it

This shrimp and broccoli dish is cheap, quick, and simple to make. It is also exceptionally healthy and is very high in protein, making it yet another perfect meal to prepare your body for long fasts.

Nutrition facts

Servings: 4

Carbs: 16 g

Protein: 29.2 g

Fat 8.1 g

Net carbs: 10 g

Calorie count per serving: 165

Ingredients

- rice or noodles (this depends on what you prefer)
- 1 lb large shrimp (peeled and cleaned)
- 1 green onion (sliced)
- 2 tbsp rice vinegar
- ¼ tsp kosher salt
- 4 tbsp soy sauce
- 1 white onion (small)
- 2 tbsp sesame oil
- ½ tbsp chili garlic (optional)
- 3 large broccoli heads
- sesame seeds to garnish

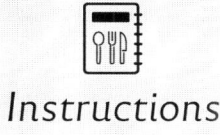

Instructions

1. Firstly, start by defrosting the shrimp (if you are unsure, check the package instructions). Generally, you can just leave them out to thaw for a while—away from your cat!
2. Chop up the broccoli heads and the onion, making sure the onion is cut into wide slices and the broccoli heads are small.
3. Take a mixing bowl and combine the chili garlic, vinegar, and soy sauce.
4. Grab a wok or a skillet and set it on medium heat.
5. Once hot, you can add the sesame oil into the pan, along with the broccoli heads, salt, and onion.
6. Cook this mixture for five to six minutes and stir often (you'll know the broccoli is ready once they are soft to the touch).
7. Toss in the shrimp for an additional three to four minutes and stir often.
8. Once ready, throw in the sauce and cook for an additional one minute.
9. Sprinkle some sesame seeds on top and enjoy!

DELICIOUS VEGGIE AND HUMMUS SANDWICH

Cooking time: 10 minutes

This vegetarian-friendly, anti-aging, heart-healthy, and dairy-free meal is perfect for a quick, convenient lunch and it's extremely good for your overall health. Plus, this sandwich is super quick and easy to make. Sometimes we overlook the simplest of meals, and these are very often the tastiest! The great thing about this meal is that you can make it in the morning or the night before in preparation for the next day, and you can carry it with you wherever you go with very little mess or fuss.

Why We Love it

Nutrition facts

Servings: 1
Carbs: 39.7 g
Protein: 12.8 g
Fat: 14.3 g
Net carbs: 28 g
Calorie count per serving: 325

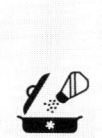
Ingredients

- 2 slices of bread (whole grain)
- 3 tbsp hummus
- ¼ cup sliced cucumber
- ¼ cup carrot (shredded)
- ¼ avocado (mashed)
- ¼ bell pepper
- ½ cup mixed greens salad

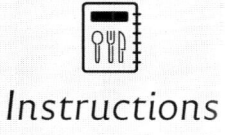
Instructions

1. Take a slice of bread and spread it evenly with hummus.
2. Take the second slice and spread it evenly with the mashed avocado.
3. Next, load the sandwich with carrot, peppers, salad greens, and cucumber.
4. You can refrigerate the sandwich for a few hours if you wish to prepare it in the morning for later on in the day, or you can enjoy it immediately.

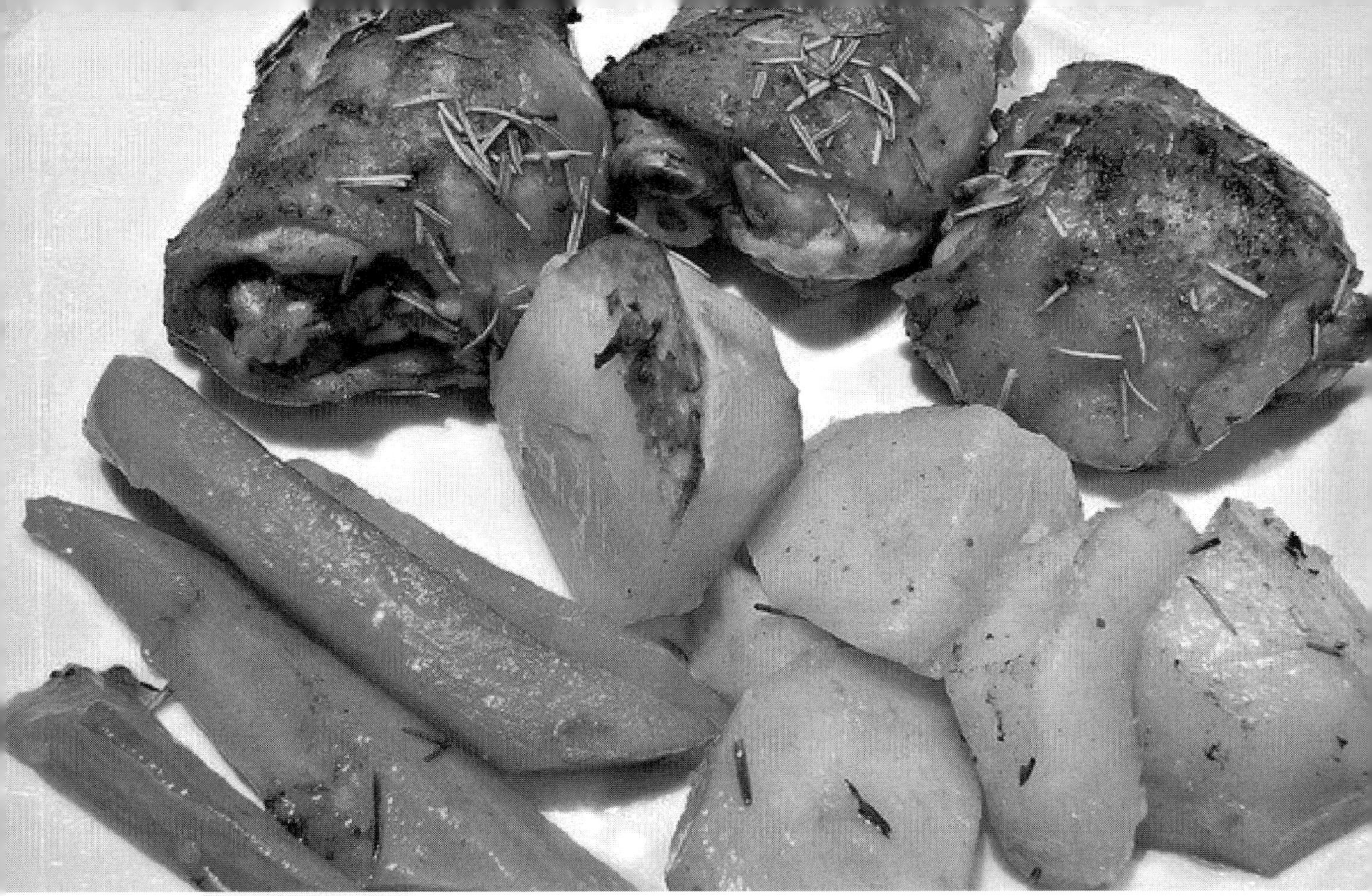

ROAST CHICKEN AND SWEET POTATOES

Cooking time: 10 minutes

Why We Love it

This next recipe is one of my favorites. There is nothing better than tender, flavorful chicken and soft sweet potatoes, especially when you know the meal is guilt-free! This recipe is a classic, and it's incredibly simple to prepare for lunch or dinner. The sweet potato is an excellent substitute for white potatoes, and it has a sweeter, more vibrant flavor.

Nutrition facts

Servings: 1

Carbs: 33.5 g

Protein: 26.9 g

Fat 17.4 g

Net carbs: 28 g

Calorie count per serving: 490

Ingredients

- 2 medium sweet potatoes (peeled and sliced into thin pieces)
- 1½ chicken thighs (skin removed)
- 2 tbsp dijon mustard
- ½ tsp salt
- 1 red onion (large)
- 2 tbsp extra virgin olive oil
- 2 tbsp fresh thyme (chopped)
- ½ tsp freshly ground pepper
- 2 cups of mixed veg (your choice)

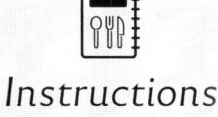

Instructions

1. Preheat the oven to 450 °F and set your oven rack to the bottom third level of the oven .
2. Next, line your tray with a rimmed baking sheet.
3. Mix together the salt, half of the oil, thyme, mustard, and pepper into a small bowl.
4. Once you have combined the ingredients thoroughly, you can marinate the chicken in the sauce.
5. Next, place the sweet potatoes and onion into a bowl and add in the rest of the oil, salt, and pepper.
6. In the meantime, remove the baking sheet from the oven and toss your vegetables of choice and potato onto the tray, spreading them evenly across the surface.
7. Next, place the marinated chicken pieces on top of the vegetables, and place the tray back into the oven for 45 minutes.
8. After approximately 20 minutes you can take the tray out and turn the vegetables over (they should be soft and tender).
9. Once the time is up you can remove the tray, dish up your food, and enjoy it while it's hot!

LAMB CHOPS WITH WILD RICE AND QUINOA

Cooking time: 3 hours 20 minutes

If there is one thing I love in this world, it's tender, tasty lamb. This next dish combines lamb with just the right amount of complex carbs to guide you through your next fast. If you're looking for a healthy dose of protein and satiety, then this is the meal to go for. In fact, this meal is perfect for someone following The Warrior Diet, as it provides you with enough calories, nutrients, and sustenance so that you don't find yourself eating too few calories throughout the day.

Why We Love it

Nutrition facts

Servings: 1

Carbs: 60 g

Protein: 26.9 g

Fat: 82.16 g

Net carbs: 55 g

Calorie count per serving: 1421

Ingredients

- 5 oz wild rice
- 5 oz quinoa
- ¾ tsp of ginger
- 12 sweet potatoes
- 12 lamb cutlets
- 1 tsp ground cumin
- 1 tsp ground paprika
- 1 tsp fresh lemon zest
- 1 pinch salt and pepper
- 5 oz feta
- 4 tbsp olive oil
- 2 freshly chopped mint sprigs
- 2 garlic cloves
- 4 scallions
- ½ tsp cayenne pepper

Instructions

1. Peel the ginger and grate it into very small pieces.
2. Next, combine the paprika, lemon zest, cumin, lemon juice, olive oil, and cayenne pepper in a bowl.
3. Prepare the lamb by rinsing and patting it dry, then coat it in the marinade and place it in the fridge for two hours.
4. After the two hours are nearly up, you can preheat the oven to 375°F.
5. Next, peel and slice the sweet potatoes and lay them out on a baking sheet.
6. Drizzle the potatoes with 2 tbsp of oil and place them in the oven for approximately 25 minutes.
7. While you wait, boil the wild rice in salted water until it is tender.
8. Place the quinoa in salted water and set the stove on high to boil for ten minutes.
9. Drain the rice and quinoa in a colander once it's ready.
10. Rinse the spinach and toss it in with the wild rice and quinoa.
11. Grab a pan and heat the remaining oil.
12. Chop and peel the garlic, then quickly rinse the scallions.
13. Dice the scallions into small pieces, then sautée them together with the garlic for a few minutes until the aromatics become fragrant.
14. Next, add the mixture of rice, quinoa, and potatoes, and combine gently.
15. Drizzle the feta and mint over top, adding some lemon juice, salt, and pepper for flavor.
16. Finally, cook the lamb on the oven griddle for approximately six to seven minutes if you prefer medium rare and make sure you cook them evenly on each side.
17. Season your juicy, tender chops with salt and pepper and toss them onto your bed of wild rice and quinoa—Enjoy!

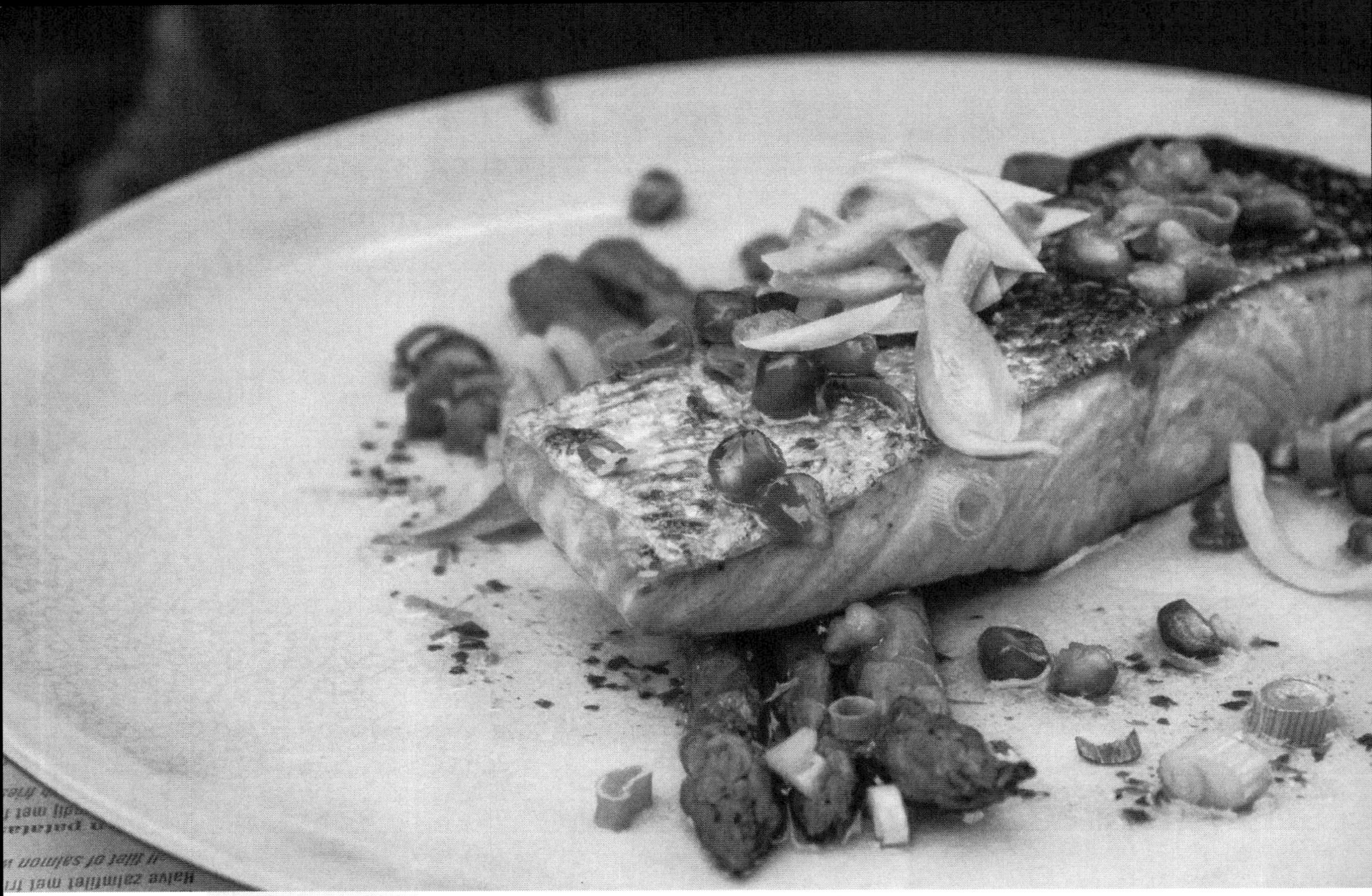

BUTTER BAKED SALMON AND ASPARAGUS

Cooking time: 30 minutes

Why We Love it

You can't get much healthier than this option! While it is normally customary to grill this combination, baking helps to draw in the healthy omega 3s that your body needs to remain young and healthy. This meal may be high in fats, but it's high in all the fats that your body needs and it's incredibly tasty.

Nutrition facts

Servings: 2
Carbs: 0 g
Protein: 26 g
Fat 52 g
Net carbs: 0 g
Calorie count per serving: 586

Ingredients

- 2 4 oz salmon fillets
- 3 tbsp butter
- 1 tbsp green onion (chopped)
- ⊠ cup mayonnaise
- 2 tbsp parsley (chopped)
- 1 tsp lemon juice
- ⊠ tsp black pepper
- ¼ tsp salt
- ½ lb asparagus (trimmed)
- ¼ tsp shredded lemon peel (optional)

Instructions

1. Start by preheating the oven to 400 °F.
2. In a saucepan, melt the butter over medium heat.
3. Next, take the salmon fillets with the skin facing downward on a baking sheet and toss the asparagus on either side, evenly drizzling the melted butter over the asparagus and salmon.
4. Sprinkle the salt and pepper over the salmon and asparagus.
5. Leave the food to bake in the oven for approximately 15 minutes (the asparagus should be soft and tender and the salmon should flake with a fork).
6. In the meantime, grab a small bowl for the garnish and mix the green onion, mayonnaise, lemon juice, lemon peel, and parsley.
7. Once the salmon and asparagus is fully cooked you can remove them from the oven and serve with your garnish.
8. Feel free to add more spices and parsley if needed and enjoy!

GNOCCHI SKILLET WITH CHICKEN SAUSAGE AND TOMATOES

Cooking time: 10-15 minutes

Why We Love it

This tasty sausage dish has less than 3 grams of fat, making it the perfect meal for trimming down. This meal is perfect for any occasion and it's rich in flavor and texture. Plus, it will only take you 10-15 minutes to whip up, making it the perfect summer meal after a relaxing day in the sun.

Nutrition facts

Servings: 4

Carbs: 90 g

Protein: 12.5 g

Fat: 2.5 g

Net carbs: 85 g

Calorie count per serving: 235

Ingredients

- 1 lb gnocchi
- 9 oz. chicken sausage (cooked) sliced into coins
- salt and pepper to taste
- 2 oz sliced basil leaves (fresh)
- 1 pint of cherry tomatoes sliced in half

Instructions

1. Grab a large pot and fill it with salted water; set it to boil on the stove over medium to high heat.
2. Toss in the gnocchi and cook for two minutes, then, once cooked, drain the gnocchi and drizzle some olive oil on top.
3. Heat up a large iron skillet over medium heat and lightly drizzle some olive oil.
4. Toss in the sausages and cook for two to three minutes, or until the sausages turn brown.
5. Move the sausages to one side of the pan and crank the heat up to high.
6. Once the skillet has reached a high heat you can throw in the cherry tomatoes and cook for one to two minutes.
7. Combine the sausage with the tomato until both are slightly blistered for a further two minutes.
8. Next, stir in the gnocchi and cook until all of the ingredients have combined (make sure that the tomatoes do not dissolve into the sauce).
9. Take the skillet off the stove and add the basil to the mix, then season with salt and pepper—Enjoy!

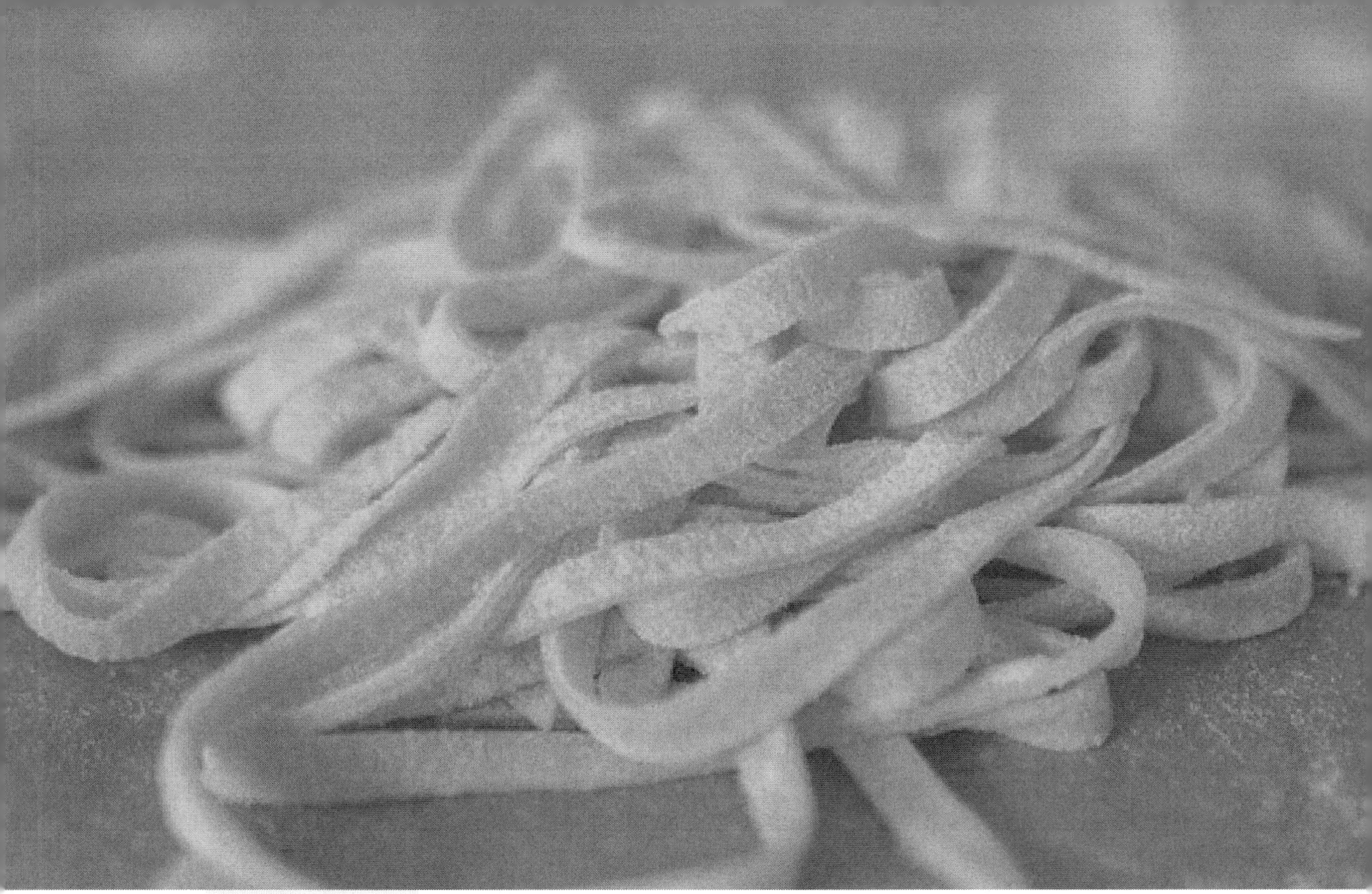

FETTUCINI CARBONARA WITH GREEN BEANS

Cooking time: 30 minutes

Why We Love it

If you're craving some carbs after a long fast, then this next meal is the perfect balance of healthy and satisfaction. The best part about this recipe is that it's not too rich or overwhelming. Plus, it only contains 360 calories which are surprisingly low for such a tasty, satisfying dish.

Nutrition facts

Servings: 4
Carbs: 65 g
Protein: 16 g

Fat: 5 g
Net carbs: 58 g
Calorie count per serving: 360

Ingredients

- 1 medium onion (chopped)
- 8 oz fettuccine
- 2 large eggs
- salt and black pepper to taste
- 4 strips of bacon (thick cut)
- parmesan
- 1 large cup of green beans

Instructions

1. To begin, start by boiling a pot of salted water on the stove.
2. In the meantime, heat a large skillet on medium and cook the bacon until crisp, then remove to drain any excess grease and place on a cutting board to be sliced into 1 1/2 inch pieces once the bacon has cooled down.
3. Next, drain the bacon fat except for approximately two tbsp from the pan and place it back on the stove, setting the heat to medium.
4. Cook the onion in the pan for five minutes until soft, allowing it to soak in the fat.
5. Once the pot of water has boiled, you can toss in the fettuccini.
6. In the meantime, add the beans to the onions and stir, tossing in some salt and pepper.
7. Leave the beans and onions to cook for about three minutes and stir occasionally.
8. While you wait for the beans and onions to cook, grab a small bowl and crack the two eggs, stirring a generous helping of black pepper into the mix. Once done, set this mixture aside for later.
9. Next, crank the heat down on the skillet to low so you don't burn the onions and beans; set them aside once they are cooked.
10. By now, your fettucini should be soft and ready (if not, wait a few more minutes).
11. Once ready, toss the fettucini into the skillet with the beans, egg mixture, and onions, and mix together thoroughly.
12. Finally, transfer the pasta into a serving bowl, season if need be, and enjoy your delicious meal!

SESAME CHICKEN

Cooking time: 35 minutes

This oriental-inspired dish is super simple to make and delicious. While your typical takeout meal similar to this one would pack close to 1,000 calories and tons of sodium, this dish contains less than half when you make it at home. It's also extremely high in protein and relatively low in carbs, making it a good option for days where you need to cut down on the carbs and ramp up the protein.

Why We Love it

Nutrition facts

Servings: 4

Carbs: 27 g

Protein: 52.8 g (without rice)

Fat: 2.5 g

Net carbs: 26.3 g

Calorie count per serving: 435

Ingredients

- 3 tbsp flour
- 2 lbs chopped chicken filets (boneless)
- 1 tbsp white vinegar
- 1 tbsp brown sugar
- 1 tbsp olive oil
- ½ tsp salt
- ½ tsp pepper
- brown rice and veg of choice
- 2 tbsp sesame oil (toasted)
- 2 minced garlic cloves
- 1 tbsp low-sodium soy sauce
- ½ cup chicken stock
- 3 tbsp toasted sesame seeds

Instructions

1. Start by preheating the oven to 400 °F.
2. Grab a small bowl and combine the chicken stock, soy sauce, sesame oil, brown sugar, vinegar, and garlic cloves.
3. While waiting for the oven, grab a large skillet and warm it up on a medium-high setting.
4. Place the chicken, salt, flour, and pepper into a bowl and toss until the chicken is covered.
5. Pour 1 tbsp of olive oil and 1 tbsp of sesame oil into the skillet.
6. Once the oils have heated in the skillet you can toss in the chicken.
7. For the next three minutes toss the chicken so that each side is evenly cooked and golden brown.
8. Next, pour the chicken stock mixture over the chicken and flip them so that both sides are covered.
9. Turn the heat off and remove the skillet, placing it in the oven for approximately 20 minutes.
10. Once baked, take the chicken out of the oven and sprinkle the sesame seeds evenly.
11. Serve the chicken with sides of your choice.

SKILLET CHIPOTLE CHICKEN ENCHILADA BAKE

Cooking time: 30-50 minutes

Why We Love it

This warm, creamy, and satisfying meal is not only low in calories but will keep you satisfied for hours to come. This is a perfect dinner option for the entire family, and the chicken and beans will help keep you feeling fuller for longer making fasting easier than ever before.

Nutrition facts

Servings: 6
Carbs: 29 g
Protein: 34.7 g
Fat: 13.6 g
Net carbs: 24 g
Calorie count per serving: 438

Ingredients

- 1 jar of green chiles
- 3 halved chicken breasts
- 1 cup of black beans
- 1 cup corn
- 1 12 oz jar Old El Paso Enchilada Sauce
- 6 tortillas
- 2 chipotle peppers (chopped)

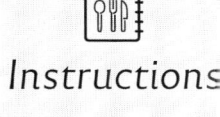

Instructions

1. Mix the chipotle peppers, chicken, enchilada sauce, and green chilies in a large pot over medium heat and combine the ingredients throughout.
2. Allow the above ingredients to cook for 20 minutes and then take the chicken out of the pot, using a fork to shred the chicken.
3. Preheat the oven to 375 °F.
4. Grab a medium-sized skillet and start to layer the ingredients in order, starting with the sauce, three tortillas, then ½ of the chicken, ½ black beans, ½ corn, and then ½ of the cheese.
5. Repeat the above step for the remaining layers.
6. Bake for the next 20-30 minutes without covering. You will know it is almost ready when the cheese starts to melt, brown, and bubble on the top.
7. As an option, you can use scallions as toppings. Enjoy!

STEAK AND BROCCOLI PROTEIN POT

Cooking time: 20 minutes

This dish comes with a massive protein punch with juicy, succulent steak, tender broccoli, ginger, and wholegrain rice. It will only take you 20 minutes to whip up, making it the perfect meal for a busy schedule.

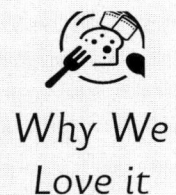

Why We Love it

Nutrition facts

Servings: 2
Carbs: 38 g
Protein: 30 g
Fat: 10 g
Net carbs: 29 g
Calorie count per serving: 385

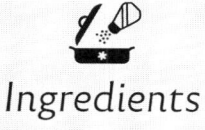

Ingredients

- One 8 oz steak filet (lean)
- 2 tbsp sushi ginger (sliced)
- 6 oz wholegrain rice
- 5.6 oz broccoli florets
- 4 spring onions (white halved lengthwise and green section chopped finely)
- 4 tbsp water

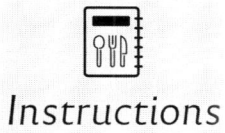

Instructions

1. Grab a large bowl and toss in the green onions, ginger, and water, along with the rice mixture.
2. Toss in the onion whites and the broccoli, making sure to keep the onions together near the surface as you will require them later.
3. Seal the bowl with some cling wrap and place in the microwave for five minutes.
4. In the meantime, set a pot of water to boil with a pinch of salt, adding in the rice to cook.
5. While you wait for the microwave and rice, grab a frying pan and set it to medium; throw in your steak, cooking it for two minutes on each side.
6. Next, toss the onion whites into the pan with the steak and allow the juices to mix for a couple of minutes.
7. Finally, pour the rice mixture into a serving bowl and add the sliced steak and cooked onions on the top.
8. Enjoy!

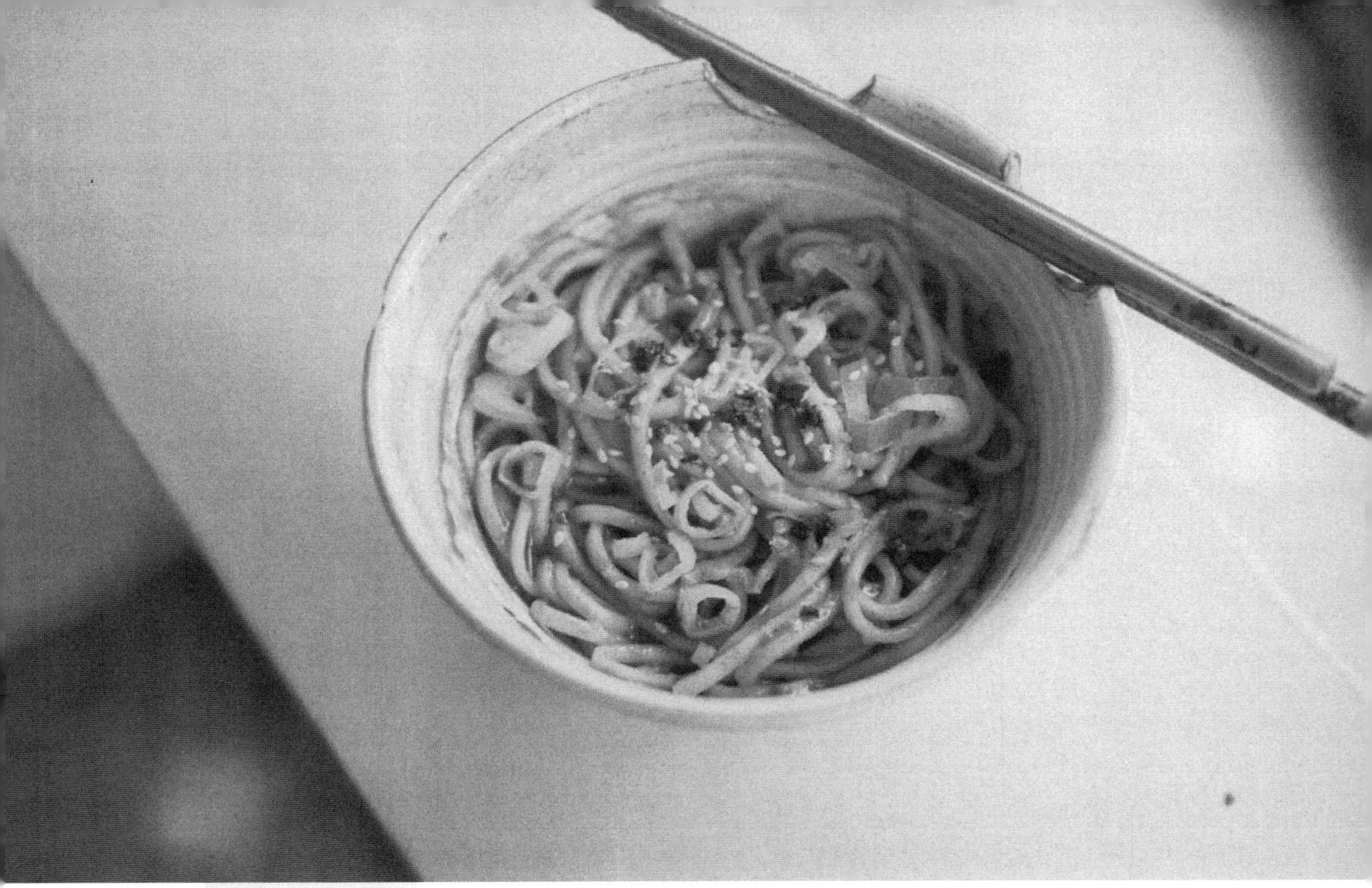

QUICK PEANUT NOODLES

Cooking time: 12 minutes

Why We Love it

One thing that I adore about stir fry is the fact that it is so quick and easy to prepare, plus it is so delicious! You can do so many things with it, including making a scrumptious peanut sauce that will have your taste buds jumping for joy! And the best part? This dish will only take you 12 minutes to prepare.

Nutrition facts

Servings: 6
Carbs: 51 g
Protein: 19.6 g
Fat 11.3 g
Net carbs: 45 g
Calorie count per serving: 380

Ingredients

- ½ cup rice vinegar
- 1 minced green onion
- 12 oz pasta (whole wheat)
- 4 green onions (minced)
- 3 tbsp peanut butter
- ¼ tbsp chopped parsley
- 1 cup mushrooms (sliced)
- 2 cups of sugar snap peas
- 1 bell pepper (red)
- 3 tbsp soy sauce
- 3-4 tbsp water

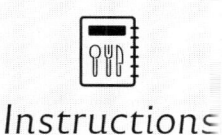

Instructions

1. Boil some water in a pot, add a pinch of salt, and toss in the pasta to cook.
2. Rinse all of your vegetables thoroughly and toss them into a wok on medium heat (excluding the cilantro).
3. Cover the vegetables and leave them to cook for several minutes.
4. While you wait you can get started on the sauce by mixing the peanut butter, green onion, soy sauce, rice vinegar, and water into a mason jar and shut the lid tightly.
5. Shake the lid as hard as you can so that the ingredients are thoroughly mixed.
6. Strain the pasta but make sure that you don't rinse it, as this will prevent the sauce from combining and sticking to the pasta (a disaster)!
7. Move the pasta into the wok with the vegetables once strained and pour in that delicious, flavorsome peanut sauce.
8. Mix everything together, take the walk off the heat, and add the cilantro.
9. Enjoy!

COD WITH CUCUMBER, AVOCADO, AND MANGO SALSA SALAD

Cooking time: 15 minutes

This quick and easy recipe is perfect for a hot summer's day and will only take you a few minutes to prepare. It's the perfect light lunch that won't leave you feeling bloated and it's full of vitamins, minerals, and antioxidants.

Why We Love it

Nutrition facts

Servings: 2

Carbs: 44.4 g

Protein: 25 g

Fat: 12 g

Net carbs: 15 g

Calorie count per serving: 272

Ingredients

- 1 small avocado (peeled, sliced, and deseeded)
- 2 spring onions
- 2 cod fillets (skinless)
- 1 handful of chopped coriander
- ¼ chopped cucumber
- 1 red chili
- 1 lime (zested)
- 5 oz cherry tomatoes
- 1 small mango peeled and sliced

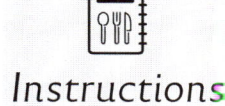
Instructions

1. Preheat your oven to 400 °F.
2. Place the cod in a shallow dish and pour half of the lime juice over top, using half of the zest and a sprinkling of ground pepper.
3. For the next eight minutes, leave the fish to bake.
4. While you wait you can toss the rest of the ingredients into a serving bowl including the rest of the lime juice.
5. Mix this combination thoroughly and then dish it up onto a plate, adding the cooked cod on top and pouring the remaining juices over top for flavor.
6. Enjoy!

TUNA NICOISE PROTEIN POT

Cooking time: 20 minutes

This next option contains a winning combination of tuna and protein, the powerhouses of energy and satiety! If you're looking for a quick on-the-go lunch, then this is the perfect option. It's also perfect for a pre or post-fast meal, as the protein will refuel your body and mind.

Why We Love it

Nutrition facts

Servings: 1
Carbs: 8 g
Protein: 30 g
Fat: 15 g
Net carbs: 4 g
Calorie count per serving: 298

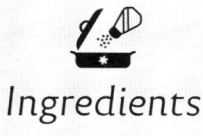
Ingredients

- 1 large egg
- 4.2 oz canned tuna
- 2.8 oz green beans
- 2 tbsp French dressing
- 1 quartered tomato

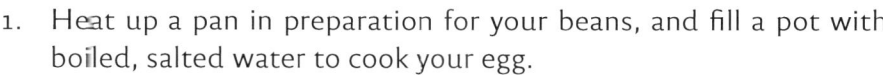

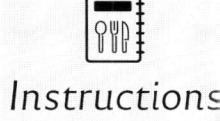
Instructions

1. Heat up a pan in preparation for your beans, and fill a pot with boiled, salted water to cook your egg.
2. Depending on how you like your egg, leave it to boil for approximately four to five minutes (longer if you like your egg hard). After five minutes your egg should be medium boiled, and the temperature of the egg should be between 180 to 190 °F.
3. While you wait, you can steam your green beans for six minutes in the pan until they turn soft.
4. Once done, you can rinse the beans and egg under cool water and set them aside to cool.
5. Next, gently peel the egg and cut it into quarters, then set aside.
6. Grab a lunch box or container and pour the beans inside, then throw your tomato, quartered egg pieces, tuna, and French dressing on top.
7. You can choose to enjoy immediately, or you can simply seal and refrigerate for later.

ORECCHIETTE WITH PEA PESTO AND WALNUTS

Cooking time: 10 minutes

This recipe is incredibly easy to make with heart-healthy, weight loss-boosting walnuts, peas, and orecchiette pasta orbs. If you're a fan of the above (and pesto, of course, then you'll love this recipe).

Why We Love it

Nutrition facts

Servings: 4

Carbs: 49.4 g

Protein: 13.3 g

Fat: 15.3 g

Net carbs: 45.4 g

Calorie count per serving: 389

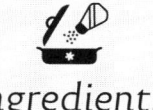
Ingredients

- 1 cup of walnuts
- 3 tsp dried Italian herbs
- ½ tbsp lemon juice
- 2 crushed garlic cloves
- 14 oz orecchiette
- 1 ½ cups peas (frozen, blanched)
- ¾ cup grated parmesan cheese
- 1 cup extra virgin olive oil

Instructions

1. All you need to do is toss the parmesan, peas, garlic, walnuts, lemon juice, and herbs into a blender and blend away.
2. In the meantime, you can cook the pasta by boiling some salted water in a pot and tossing it in.
3. Once cooked, drain the water until ½ of a cup of the boiled water is left, and then add the pasta into a serving bowl. Set the remaining boiled water aside.
4. Simply mix the pesto in with the remaining cooking water and the pasta and combine thoroughly.
5. Sprinkle walnuts on top for garnish.
6. Enjoy!

LEMON CHICKEN KEBABS WITH TOMATO AND PARSLEY SALAD

Cooking time: 2 hours 15 minutes

This protein-rich dish is perfect for a light lunch on a summer's day and won't leave you feeling bloated or uncomfortable. It's also super low in calories, meaning that you can enjoy it guilt-free!

Why We Love it

Nutrition facts

Servings: 4

Carbs: 6 g

Protein: 38 g

Fat: 8.8 g

Net carbs: 2 g

Calorie count per serving: 311

Ingredients

- 1 cup cherry tomatoes (chopped)
- 3 tbsp extra virgin olive oil
- 1 ½ tbsp oregano (dried)
- 6 oz skinless, boneless chicken breasts halved and cut into small cubes
- 3 tbsp fresh lemon juice
- ¾ tsp kosher salt
- 1 tbsp garlic (minced)
- 2 cups fresh parsley

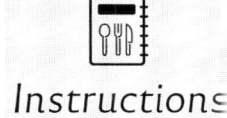
Instructions

1. Combine the lemon juice, oregano, garlic, salt, pepper, and oil into a bowl.
2. Grab a whisk and mix thoroughly, then add the chicken and place the bowl in the fridge for two hours to properly marinate.
3. Start by heating a grill pan on medium heat and remove the chicken from the marinade, tossing the excess away.
4. Place the chicken pieces onto four wooden skewers and set them on the grill, leaving them to cook for approximately six minutes (the chicken should feel tender to the touch).
5. Combine the remaining juice, garlic, oregano, salt, and pepper in a bowl.
6. Slowly combine the remaining oil into the bowl and thoroughly whisk everything together.
7. Finally, toss in the tomatoes and the parsley.
8. Add the chicken on top of the salad and dig in!

FENNEL ROASTED CHICKEN AND PEPPERS

Cooking time: 35 minutes

This lean, high-protein meal is a quick and easy dinner option to prepare you for a successful overnight fast without the cravings.

Why We Love it

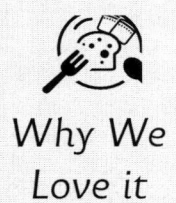

Nutrition facts

Servings: 4
Carbs: 11 g
Protein: 32 g
Fat: 40 g
Net carbs: 6 g
Calorie count per serving: 530

Ingredients

- 5 tbsp olive oil
- 6 cloves garlic (sliced)
- 1 tsp kosher salt
- 1 tbsp fennel seeds
- 1 tsp pepper
- 2 oz feta cheese (crumbled)
- 4 cups baby spinach
- 4 chicken drumsticks
- 4 (in total) sliced red, yellow, and green peppers (you can mix them together)
- 1 tbsp grated orange zest

Instructions

1. Preheat the pan to 425 °F.
2. For the next three to four minutes, cook the fennel seeds and the orange zest in a small skillet until lightly browned.
3. Next, you'll need to grind or pulse them together with a spice grinder (if you have a blender this will be the easiest method).
4. On a large baking sheet, add 4 tbsp of oil, bell peppers, and garlic to the surface.
5. Now, sprinkle ¾ tsp of the salt and pepper for flavor.
6. Transfer half of the above ingredients to the second sheet and organize them in an identical layer on each.
7. Next, marinate the chicken pieces with the remainder of the oil, fennel seed, and orange mix.
8. Place the chicken pieces over the top of the vegetables on each baking sheet and roast for approximately 20 to 30 minutes until the chicken has turned golden-brown.
9. Move the chicken from the tray to a serving plate, toss the spinach over the vegetables and mix.
10. Finally, add the vegetables and remaining salt and pepper to the chicken and garnish with feta—Enjoy!

LOW-CALORIE CHICKEN MARSALA

Cooking time: 35 minutes

Who doesn't love a good chicken marsala? This is an Italian-American dish that is not only creamy, quick, and delicious, but it's really simple to prepare at home. While some marsalas can pack a heavy calorie count, this one is calorie-conscious meaning that you can enjoy it as part of your fasting routine without feeling guilty.

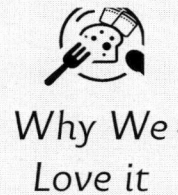

Why We Love it

Nutrition facts

Servings: 4

Carbs: 14 g

Protein: 42 g

Fat: 11 g

Net carbs: 7.6 g

Calorie count per serving: 335

Ingredients

- 3 tbsp flour
- 1 shallot
- 1 garlic clove
- 6 oz boneless chicken breast (4 of each)
- 10 oz sliced mushrooms
- ½ cup marsala wine
- ¼ tsp salt
- ¼ tsp pepper
- ½ cup chicken broth (low-sodium)

Instructions

1. Depending on what item you have at your disposal, you can use a rolling pin or the bottom of a pan to flatten the chicken filets so that they are half an inch thick.
2. Next, add some flavor by sprinkling salt and pepper on the chicken.
3. Coat the chicken in the flour, making sure to cover it evenly.
4. Grab a large skillet and heat 1 tbsp of olive oil in the pan; toss in the chicken, cooking for approximately five minutes on each side.
5. Once the chicken is cooked you can remove it from the skillet and place it on a plate.
6. Next, grate the shallot and garlic into fine pieces.
7. Using the same skillet that you cooked the chicken in, add 1 tbsp of olive oil and cook the mushrooms on medium-high heat for five minutes.
8. Make sure that you toss the mushrooms every so often so that they brown evenly on each side.
9. Once the five minutes are up you can toss in the garlic and shallots for an additional two minutes, seasoning it with the remaining salt and pepper.
10. Next, add the chicken broth and wine to the skillet with the chicken and simmer until the liquid is reduced by at least half.
11. Leave this for approximately four minutes and then garnish with the chopped parsley.
12. Finally, serve the final product with spinach and dig in!

CHICKEN BURGER WITH SUN-DRIED TOMATO

Cooking time: 20 minutes

If you're anything like me, I absolutely love my burgers! The problem is that they're generally not the healthiest options around, especially when they're made from processed beef. The good news is that chicken burgers can taste just as good when cooked properly, and they contain half the calories, which is exactly why I added it to this list.

Why We Love it

Nutrition facts

Servings: 4

Carbs: 21 g

Protein: 13 g

Fat: 14 g

Net carbs: 7 g

Calorie count per serving: 330

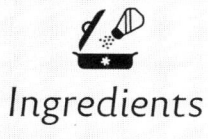
Ingredients

- 1 lb lean chicken breast
- 2 cups baby spinach, arugula, or any mixed greens of your choice
- salt and pepper to taste
- juice from half a lemon
- 1 tsp fresh rosemary
- 2 tbsp olive oil mayo
- 2 tbsp sun-dried tomatoes (chopped)
- 2 cloves finely sliced garlic
- 4 buns (whole wheat)

Instructions

1. Grab a bowl and toss in the mayo, garlic, rosemary, sun-dried tomatoes, and lemon juice for the marinade and set aside for later.
2. Next, preheat a skillet or grill depending on what you have available.
3. Throw in some oil into the pan (if you are using a skillet) in preparation for the chicken and wait for it to heat up on medium-high.
4. Next, gently mold the chicken into four evenly sized patties.
5. Once the pan is hot, you can toss in the chicken patties with black pepper and salt (if you are using a grill you can simply place the chicken patties straight on to cook).
6. For the next five or six minutes, cook the patties until they have browned and turned slightly crisp, then flip them over for an additional three to four minutes
7. Next, toast the buns so that they are crisp and fresh.
8. Once the patties are ready, remove them from the heat and set them aside.
9. Now, you need to cover the chicken with the aioli that you prepared earlier, which is essentially a mixture of garlic and olive oil (super tasty and much healthier than other alternatives).
10. Layer the buns with your choice of greens and place the patty on the top, pour the sauces, and top with the bun—Enjoy!

CONCLUSION

While this may be the last section of the book, this is only the first page of your chapter. The biggest questions that women—especially mature ladies—have to ask about IF is whether it is effective and why it works? In this book, you've learned that IF can be an exceptionally effective tool, not only for weight loss, but for longevity, disease management and prevention, and mental clarity.

There's also a spiritual side to fasting, as it prompts you to be more in touch with your body and mind, by eating mindfully and taking note of your hunger signals, urges, and emotions. With all this in mind, it's really important that you do pay careful attention to your body's signals when you fast. If fasting is making you really sick or you're feeling terrible, then you may want to try an alternative weight-loss method. That said, most women have no issues and find that IF has changed their lives for the better in several ways.

Now that you're at the end of this book you're probably dying to start preparing your new list of recipes, but you're probably also wondering how important calorie-counting is. When it comes to IF, the main focus is *when* you eat rather than *what* you eat; however, you're not doing your health any favors by eating processed foods with very little nutritional value and more calories than they're worth. After all, wouldn't you rather eat *more* food, feel more energized, and see quicker results? If the answer is yes, then make the effort to follow the above recipes and prepare wholesome, home-cooked meals for yourself and your family. Plus, your complexion, hair, and waistline will reflect your culinary efforts!

I didn't write this book to emphasize the importance of being slim and reaching for perfection—I wrote it to help older women feel better not only on the outside but on the *inside*. Once you change your lifestyle, your way of thinking, your relationship with food, and your body, everything else falls into place. If you walk into a new way of eating with the sole intention of losing weight, you're missing the bigger picture. Weight loss is only one of the many benefits of IF, but personally, I find that challenging your mind, willpower, and changing old, toxic habits is the biggest achievement.

If you're feeling nervous about this new journey (which is perfectly normal, by the way), just remember that slow and steady wins the race. Just to reiterate, always start with a short fast and work your way up to longer increments. In fact, spontaneously skipping a meal here and there is also a great way to start, as you can successfully gauge how your body reacts to a missed meal, and this can help to prepare you for your first proper fast. Once you've successfully done this, you can move on to fasting for 12 hours for a couple of days per week, then gradually increase the hours and days as you feel more comfortable. Make sure that you are drinking plenty of water, and do your absolute best to stick to wholesome, nutrient-dense home-cooked meals to fuel your body and promote faster weight loss.

Once you develop a routine you can start to seriously decide which fasting method you want to follow. This will depend on a variety of factors, namely: your work schedule, family, social calendar, and general preferences. The great thing about IF is that you can play around with different methods until you find one that fits your lifestyle best. Don't feel chained to just one method if you feel that it isn't working for you, branch out and find something new!

Another important take-home point is to keep track of your progress. Keep a journal and write down your physical and mental symptoms so that you can identify triggers and behaviors that either hinder or boost your progress. For example, which emotions or habits have caused you to break your fast, or which activities helped you to stick to it? Start to notice patterns and identify the negatives so that you can avoid them in the future.

Also remember to find a strong support system, whether your loved ones join you or simply hold your hand through the journey. If you feel that you won't receive that support, then don't feel the need to share anything and stick with your decision. There are tons of IF support groups on social media sites such as Facebook, where members can discuss their experiences and provide advice for those in need. Embarking on such a big change in your lifestyle can be frustrating and emotional in the beginning, which is why you need support. The good news is that it's only short-lived and you'll be better off and healthier as a result!

So, What Next?

By now you're probably tired of reading, so it's time to get out there and make that change! The first thing you'll need to do is create a shopping list of all the ingredients you'll need to make the above-mentioned recipes. Secondly, (this isn't mandatory, but I recommend it) you need to throw out any tempting foods: chocolates, cakes, cookies, and chips should not be staring you in the face every time you enter your kitchen!

Once you've prepared your meal and decided on your method, it's time to tell your friends and family (if you feel they will be supportive) and get started. You can also buy yourself a pretty journal to motivate you and track your information, download a good tracking application for your progress, and get excited!

Also (and this is so important) be kind to yourself. There are going to be days where you feel overwhelmed, disheartened, and ready to give up the battle. That said, these are the days that you need to fight the hardest! Understand that there will be days when you mess up, and that is perfectly okay. We are all human, and sometimes you need to fall off the wagon to get right back on. You can expect to make a few slip-ups in the first few days of your fasting experience, so don't allow that to cause you to give up altogether.

Most importantly, don't allow fasting to take over your life and take over social commitments, family time, or your health. If you ever have to skip a family breakfast with a loved one for a fast, then you're overdoing it. Remember, if you miss a fasting day, there's always tomorrow. You can relive the fasting experience but you cannot do the same with an experience with someone you care about.

Lastly, and most importantly, please feel free to leave a review on this book.

Scan the QR code:

Experts are still debating many aspects of intermittent fasting despite numerous studies, and this book has summarized all of the most relevant and up-to-date information that you will need to progress on this journey. That said, I'm always open to suggestions and improvement and we are still learning new things every day when it comes to nutrition and health. Hopefully, in the future, experts will perform more studies on the effects of fasting in humans so that we can fully understand the remarkable effects of fasting on the body.

I trust you will experience excellent health and well-being on the long road of life that lies before you and wish you my very best. Thank you for letting me share my knowledge with you.

Britney Lynch

REFERENCES

12 Tips to Achieve Fasting Success - Personal Excellence. Personal Excellence. (2021). https://personalexcellence.co/blog/fasting-success/.

A Fasting Diet Shouldn't Turn You Into A Hangry Betch—Here's How To Do It Right. Women's Health. (2021). https://www.womenshealthmag.com/weight-loss/a29602869/fasting-tips/.

A Flavor-Packed, Warm Kale-Quinoa Salad Recipe | Eat This Not That. (2021). https://www.eatthis.com/kale-quinoa-salad/.

Add Flavor to Your Night With This Fennel Roasted Chicken and Peppers Dinner. Good Housekeeping. (2018). https://www.goodhousekeeping.com/food-recipes/easy/a25656846/fennel-roasted-chicken-and-peppers-recipe/.

Bagherniya, M., Butler, A., Barreto, G., & Sahebkar, A. (2018). The effect of fasting or calorie restriction on autophagy induction: A review of the literature. *Ageing Research Reviews*, *47*, 183-197. https://doi.org/10.1016/j.arr.2018.08.004

Banana-Flax Breakfast Muffins. Vegetarian Times. (2021). https://www.vegetariantimes.com/recipes/banana-flax-breakfast-muffins/.

Bellisle, F., McDevitt, R., & Prentice, A. (1997). Meal frequency and energy balance. *British Journal Of Nutrition*, *77*(S1), S57-S70. https://doi.org/10.1079/bjn19970104

Bredesen, D. (2014). Reversal of cognitive decline: A novel therapeutic program. *Aging*, *6*(9), 707-717. https://doi.org/10.18632/aging.100690

Buckingham, C. (2020). *11 People Who Should Never Try Intermittent Fasting | Eat This Not That*. https://www.eatthis.com/is-intermittent-fasting-safe/.

Buenfeld, S. (2021). *Spicy Chicken & Avocado Wraps Recipe | BBC Good Food*.

Bbcgoodfood.com. https://www.bbcgoodfood.com/recipes/spicy-chicken-avocado-wraps.

Buenfeld, S. (2021). *Steak & Broccoli Protein Pots Recipe | BBC Good Food.* Bbcgoodfood.com. https://www.bbcgoodfood.com/recipes/steak-broccoli-protein-pots.

Buenfeld, S. (2021). *Tuna Niçoise Protein Pot Recipe | BBC Good Food.* Bbcgoodfood.com. https://www.bbcgoodfood.com/recipes/tuna-nicoise-protein-pots.

Calabrese, E. (2021). *Caprese Zoodles. Delish.* https://www.delish.com/cooking/recipe-ideas/recipes/a47336/caprese-zoodles-recipe/.

Cherrier, C. (2021). *Lemon Garlic Butter Chicken Thighs and Green Beans Skillet.* Eatwell101. https://www.eatwell101.com/lemon-garlic-butter-thighs-and-green-beans-skillet.

Chicken Marsala. Good Housekeeping. (2021). https://www.goodhousekeeping.com/food-recipes/easy/a47886/chicken-marsala-recipe/.

Clark, E. (2020). *Meatball & Tomato Soup Recipe | BBC Good Food.* Bbcgoodfood.com. https://www.bbcgoodfood.com/recipes/meatball-tomato-soup.

Cod with Cucumber, Avocado & Mango Salsa Salad Recipe | BBC Good Food. Bbcgoodfood.com. (2021). https://www.bbcgoodfood.com/recipes/cod-cucumber-avocado-mango-salsa-salad.

Cohen, M. (2020). *The 7 Best Apps for Intermittent Fasting.* Good Housekeeping. https://www.goodhousekeeping.com/health-products/g34618367/best-apps-intermittent-fasting/.

Cousineau, R. (2021). *Lemony Chicken Kebabs with Tomato-Parsley Salad Recipe.* MyRecipes. https://www.myrecipes.com/recipe/lemony-chicken-kebabs-tomato-parsley-salad.

Coyle, D. (2017). *7 Foods That Still Contain Trans Fats.* Healthline. https://www.healthline.com/nutrition/trans-fat-foods

Coyle, D. (2018). *Intermittent Fasting For Women: A Beginner's Guide.* Healthline. https://www.healthline.com/nutrition/intermittent-fasting-for-women.

Coyle, D. (2020). *Everything You Want to Know About the Low Glycemic Diet.* Healthline. https://www.healthline.com/nutrition/low-glycemic-diet#foods-to-eat.

Dalkin, G. (2015). *Skillet Chipotle Chicken Enchilada Bake - What's Gaby Cooking*. What's Gaby Cooking. https://whatsgabycooking.com/skillet-chipotle-chicken-enchilada-bake/.

Davis, C. P. (2021, March 22). *How Long Do You Need to Fast for Autophagy?* MedicineNet. https://www.medicinenet.com/how_long_do_you_need_to_fast_for_autophagy/article.htm

de Groot, S., Pijl, H., van der Hoeven, J. J. M., & Kroep, J. R. (2019). Effects of short-term fasting on cancer treatment. *Journal of Experimental & Clinical Cancer Research, 38*(1). https://doi.org/10.1186/s13046-019-1189-9

Dhurandhar, E. J., Dawson, J., Alcorn, A., Larsen, L. H., Thomas, E. A., Cardel, M., Bourland, A. C., Astrup, A., St-Onge, M.-P., Hill, J. O., Apovian, C. M., Shikany, J. M., & Allison, D. B. (2014). The effectiveness of breakfast recommendations on weight loss: a randomized controlled trial. *The American Journal of Clinical Nutrition, 100*(2), 507–513. https://doi.org/10.3945/ajcn.114.089573

Doherty, C. (2020). *How Fasting Causes Headaches*. Verywell Health. https://www.verywellhealth.com/how-fasting-can-cause-a-headache-1719448.

Drop in Both Insulin and Leptin Needed for Fat Burning to Occur - Diabetes. Diabetes. (2018). https://www.diabetes.co.uk/news/2018/jan/drop-in-both-insulin-and-leptin-needed-for-fat-burning-to-occur-90969878.html.

Durand, F. (2021). *Gnocchi Skillet with Chicken Sausage & Tomatoes*. Eat This, Not That. https://www.thekitchn.com/recipe-gnocchi-skillet-with-chicken-sausage-amp-tomatoes-206420

Eenfeldt, A. Dr. (2020). *Intermittent Fasting in Women Over 60 – Diet Doctor*. Diet Doctor. https://www.dietdoctor.com/intermittent-fasting-in-women-over-60.

Entin, E. (2015). *Stop Eating...Until Tomorrow*. The Doctor Will See You Now. http://www.thedoctorwillseeyounow.com/content/cancer/art4652.html.

Fasting can slow down ageing! - Times of India. The Times of India. (2020). https://timesofindia.indiatimes.com/life-style/food-news/can-fasting-slow-down-aging/articleshow/73057733.cms.

Geimer, P. (2021). *Anti-Inflammatory Superfood Turmeric Berry Smoothie*. Further Food. https://www.furtherfood.com/recipe/anti-inflammatory-superfood-turmeric-berries-smoothie-daily-turmeric-tonic/.

Getting Started with Intermittent Fasting - My Tips for an Easy Transition. Pure Health Transitions. (2021). Retrieved 3 August 2021, from https://purehealthtransitions.com/getting-started-with-intermittent-fasting/.

Gunnars, K. (2017). *What Is Intermittent Fasting? Explained in Human Terms*. Healthline. https://www.healthline.com/nutrition/what-is-intermittent-fasting.

Gunnars, K. (2021). *10 Health Benefits of Intermittent Fasting*. Healthlinehttps://www.healthline.com/nutrition/10-health-benefits-of-intermittent-fasting.

Gunnars, K. (2019). 1*1 Myths About Fasting and Meal Frequency*. Healthline. https://www.healthline.com/nutrition/11-myths-fasting-and-meal-frequency.

Heffernan, C. (2020). *Guest Post: The History of Intermittent Fasting - Physical Culture Study*. Physical Culture Study. https://physicalculturestudy.com/2020/04/21/guest-post-the-history-of-intermittent-fasting/.

Hodgkin, E. (2017). *The warrior diet: Plan including fasting and intensive exercise NOT for the faint hearted*. Express.co.uk. https://www.express.co.uk/life-style/diets/755630/warrior-diet-plan.

Honey Mustard Pork Chops and Potato Skillet. Eatwell101. (2021). https://www.eatwell101.com/honey-mustard-pork-chops-and-potatoes-recipe#recipecardo.

Horton, B. (2021). *Should You Try Eat-Stop-Eat to Lose Weight? | Livestrong.com*. LIVESTRONG.COM. https://www.livestrong.com/article/438695-how-eat-stop-eat-works/.

https://pixabay.com/photos/breakfast-acai-bowl-breakfast-bowl-5551495/

https://pixabay.com/photos/fettuccine-pasta-flour-noodles-5992799/

https://pixabay.com/photos/girl-woman-people-holding-yogurt-791563/

https://pixabay.com/photos/lamb-lamb-chop-flesh-grilling-meal-1095653/

https://pixabay.com/photos/lentil-soup-food-meal-yummy-2325144/

https://pixabay.com/photos/roasted-chicken-thighs-potatoes-1005314/

https://pixabay.com/photos/shrimps-broccoli-plate-platter-5977365/

https://pixabay.com/photos/vegan-wrap-herbal-meal-healthy-946034/

https://pixabay.com/photos/woman-question-mark-person-decision-687560/

https://pixabay.com/photos/zucchini-noodle-noodles-zoodle-2340977/

https://unsplash.com/photos/bHhEJAXyFOg

https://unsplash.com/photos/FMjoqc4p8WE

https://unsplash.com/photos/kp8vmhqytuM

https://unsplash.com/photos/lJLXlh7KT38

https://unsplash.com/photos/LxC1Qx1qulc

https://unsplash.com/photos/sBOl-XPYv9M

https://unsplash.com/photos/t05q7TZObzc

https://unsplash.com/photos/XBxRJWzV8RM

https://unsplash.com/s/photos/pork-chops

https://unsplash.com/s/photos/tomato-soup

Intermittent Fasting: *What is it, and how does it work?*. (2021). https://www.hopkinsmedicine.org/health/wellness-and-prevention/intermittent-fasting-what-is-it-and-how-does-it-work.

Publishing, H. H. (2020, April 1). *Is intermittent fasting safe for older adults?* Harvard Health. https://www.health.harvard.edu/staying-healthy/is-intermittent-fasting-safe-for-older-adults

Jandial, R. (2020). *The Popular Diet One Neurosurgeon Swears By as a Way to Boost Your Brainpower*. Health.com. https://www.health.com/nutrition/brain-health-intermittent-fasting\.

Jandial, R. (2020). *The Popular Diet One Neurosurgeon Swears By as a Way to Boost Your Brainpower*. Health.com. https://www.health.com/nutrition/brain-health-intermittent-fasting\.

Johnstone, A., Faber, P., Gibney, E., Elia, M., Horgan, G., Golden, B., & Stubbs, R. (2002). Effect of an acute fast on energy compensation and feeding behaviour in lean men and women. *International Journal Of Obesity, 26*(12), 1623-1628. https://doi.

org/10.1038/sj.ijo.0802151

Kadouch, J. (2020). *The Alternate-day Fasting Guide*. Medium. https://medium.com/in-fitness-and-in-health/the-alternate-day-fasting-guide-a69a45e77473.

Kim, K., Kim, Y., Son, J., Lee, J., Kim, S., & Choe, M. et al. (2021). Intermittent fasting promotes adipose thermogenesis and metabolic homeostasis via VEGF-mediated alternative activation of macrophage. Retrieved 27 July 2021, from.

Kim, K.-H., Kim, Y. H., Son, J. E., Lee, J. H., Kim, S., Choe, M. S., Moon, J. H., Zhong, J., Fu, K., Lenglin, F., Yoo, J.-A., Bilan, P. J., Klip, A., Nagy, A., Kim, J.-R., Park, J. G., Hussein, S. M., Doh, K.-O., Hui, C., & Sung, H.-K. (2017). Intermittent fasting promotes adipose thermogenesis and metabolic homeostasis via VEGF-mediated alternative activation of macrophage. *Cell Research, 27*(11), 1309–1326. https://doi.org/10.1038/cr.2017.126

Kingsley, T. (2017, August 29). *Thai Salmon with Carrot Salad*. Further Food. https://www.furtherfood.com/recipe/thai-salmon-carrot-salad-gluten-free-paleo/

Kubala, J. (2019). *The 20 Best Ways to Lose Weight After 50*. Healthline. https://www.healthline.com/nutrition/how-to-lose-weight-after-50.

Kubala, J. (2021). *9 Potential Intermittent Fasting Side Effects*. Healthline. https://www.healthline.com/nutrition/intermittent-fasting-side-effects.

Lamb Chops with Wild Rice and Quinoa. Eat Smarter USA. (2021). https://eatsmarter.com/recipes/lamb-chops-with-wild-rice-and-quinoa.

Lederer, M. (2020). 5 Intermittent Fasting Mistakes Causing Common Side Effects. Mental Food Chain. Retrieved 20 August 2021, from https://www.mentalfoodchain.com/intermittent-fasting-side-effects/.

Legg, T. (2018). *Emotional Eating: Why It Happens and How to Stop It*. Healthline. https://www.healthline.com/health/emotional-eating.

Link, R. (2018). *16/8 Intermittent Fasting: A Beginner's Guide*. Healthline. https://www.healthline.com/nutrition/16-8-intermittent-fasting.

Longo, V., & Mattson, M. (2014). Fasting: Molecular Mechanisms and Clinical Applications. *Cell Metabolism, 19*(2), 181-192. https://doi.org/10.1016/j.cmet.2013.12.008

Longo, V., & Panda, S. (2016). Fasting, Circadian Rhythms, and Time-Restricted

Feeding in Health Lifespan. *Cell Metabolism, 23*(6), 1048-1059. https://doi.org/10.1016/j.cmet.2016.06.001

Mann, D. (2021). *What to Know About Alternate-Day Fasting Schedules.* The Healthy. https://www.thehealthy.com/weight-loss/alternate-day-fasting-schedules/.

Marengo, K. (2019). *The 5:2 diet: A guide and meal plan.* Medicalnewstoday.com. https://www.medicalnewstoday.com/articles/324303#how-to-eat-on-fast-days.

Mazzoni, M. (2021). *Ginger Maple Glazed Salmon (Dairy-Free, Gluten-Free, Low-Carb).* Further Food. https://www.furtherfood.com/recipe/ginger-maple-glazed-salmon-dairy-free-gluten-free-low-carb/.

Merchant, J. (2021). *Simple Sesame Chicken Skillet..* How Sweet Eats. https://www.howsweeteats.com/2012/10/simple-sesame-chicken-skillet/.

Metabolic switching may be the key to weight loss and good health-Health News , Firstpost. Firstpost. (2020). https://www.firstpost.com/health/metabolic-switching-may-be-the-key-to-weight-loss-and-good-health-7856721.html.

Morin, K. (2017). *5 Intermittent Fasting Methods: Which One Is Best for You?.* Life by Daily Burn. https://dailyburn.com/life/health/intermittent-fasting-methods/.

Nair, P., & Khawale, P. (2016). Role of therapeutic fasting in women's health: An overview. *Journal Of Mid-Life Health, 7*(2), 61. https://doi.org/10.4103/0976-7800.185325

Nies, N. (2021). *Acai Breakfast Bowl.* Further Food. https://www.furtherfood.com/recipe/acai-breakfast-bowl-vegan-arthritis-diet/.

Olson, A. (2014). *Peanut Stir-Fry Recipe | One Ingredient Chef.* Oneingredientchef.com. http://www.oneingredientchef.com/12-minute-peanut-noodles/.

Overhiser, S. (2021). *Best Ever Lentil Soup.* A Couple Cooks. https://www.acouplecooks.com/shrimp-and-broccoli/.

Overhiser, S. (2021). *Shrimp and Broccoli.* A Couple Cooks. https://www.acouplecooks.com/shrimp-and-broccoli/.

Parker-Pope, T. (2007). *The Risks and Rewards of Skipping Meals.* Well. https://well.blogs.nytimes.com/2007/12/26/the-risks-and-rewards-of-skipping-meals/.

Pomegranate Sunflower Yogurt Recipe. Nutritious Life: Healthy Tips, Healthy Recipes,

Exercise. (2021). from https://nutritiouslife.com/recipes/pomegranate-sunflower-yogurt/.

Rd., W. (2020). *The Truth About Autophagy : Fasting, Exercise, Coffee!* - Whitney E. RD. Whitney E. RD. https://www.whitneyerd.com/2020/01/the-truth-about-autophagy.html.

Regushadze, L. (2021). *Lemon Chicken Avocado Salad*. Further Food. https://www.furtherfood.com/recipe/lemon-chicken-avocado-salad-rosemary-wheat-berries-high-iron/.

Roast Chicken & Sweet Potatoes. EatingWell. (2021). https://www.eatingwell.com/recipe/250549/roast-chicken-sweet-potatoes/.

Sadhukhan, P. (2021). *The Warrior Diet: Results, Meal Plan, And Benefits To Lose Weight*. STYLECRAZE. https://www.stylecraze.com/articles/warrior-diet-plan-a-complete-guide/.

Stote, K., Baer, D., Spears, K., Paul, D., Harris, G., & Rumpler, W. et al. (2007). A controlled trial of reduced meal frequency without caloric restriction in healthy, normal-weight, middle-aged adults. *The American Journal Of Clinical Nutrition, 85*(4), 981-988. https://doi.org/10.1093/ajcn/85.4.981

Superfood Oatmeal Recipe. Nutritious Life: Healthy Tips, Healthy Recipes, Exercise. (2021). https://nutritiouslife.com/recipes/supercharged-oatmeal/.

Sweet Potato Chickpea Buddha Bowl. Minimalist Baker. (2021). https://minimalistbaker.com/sweet-potato-chickpea-buddha-bowl/.

Tabahlia, J. (2021). *12-Hour Intermittent Fasting For Weight Loss And Other Benefits*. BetterMe Blog. https://betterme.world/articles/12-hour-intermittent-fasting/.

Taylor, K. (2021). *Savory Steel Cut Oatmeal*. Cookie and Kate. https://cookieandkate.com/savory-steel-cut-oatmeal-recipe/.

Taylor, M. (2017). *What You Should Know About Crescendo Fasting—The Intermittent Fasting Diet For Women*. Prevention. https://www.prevention.com/weight-loss/a20493417/the-intermittent-fasting-diet-for-women/.

The Pros And Cons Of Skipping Breakfast. sheerluxe.com. (2021). https://sheerluxe.com/health-wellness/pros-and-cons-of-skipping-breakfast.

Varady, K. (2011). Intermittent versus daily calorie restriction: which diet regimen is more effective for weight loss?. *Obesity Reviews, 12*(7), e593-e601. https://doi.org/10.1111/j.1467-789x.2011.00873.x

Wallis, C. (2021). *How Good a Diet Is Intermittent Fasting?*. Scientific American. https://www.scientificamerican.com/article/how-good-a-diet-is-intermittent-fasting/.

Webster, K. (2017). *Veggie & Hummus Sandwich*. EatingWell.https://www.eatingwell.com/recipe/259887/veggie-hummus-sandwich/.

West, H. (2019). *How to Fast Safely: 10 Helpful Tips*. Healthline. https://www.healthline.com/nutrition/how-to-fast#TOC_TITLE_HDR_9.

What Is Intermittent Fasting and Does It Really Work? (2019, November 23). The New York Times. http://www.nytimes.com/2019/11/23/style/self-care/intermittent-fasting-benefits.html

What to Know About Intermittent Fasting for Women After 50. WebMD. (2021). https://www.webmd.com/healthy-aging/what-to-know-about-intermittent-fasting-for-women-after-50.

Why Is Protein Important In Your Diet? | Piedmont Healthcare. Piedmont.org. (2021). https://www.piedmont.org/living-better/why-is-protein-important-in-your-diet.

William, B. (202) *Intermittent Fasting Vs Calorie Restriction: Which Approach Can Propel Your Weight Loss Into High Gear?*. BetterMe Blog. https://betterme.world/articles/intermittent-fasting-vs-calorie-restriction/.

Winn, E. (2021). *Crustless Spinach Quiche (Dairy-Free, Paleo, Whole30)*. Further Food. https://www.furtherfood.com/recipe/crustless-spinach-quiche-dairy-free-paleo-whole30-gluten-free-high-protein/.

Wnuk, A. (2018). *How Does Fasting Affect the Brain?*. Brainfacts.org. https://www.brainfacts.org/thinking-sensing-and-behaving/diet-and-lifestyle/2018/how-does-fasting-affect-the-brain-071318.

Wood, P. (2021). *Orecchiette With Walnut and Pea Pesto*. delicious.com.au.https://www.delicious.com.au/recipes/orecchiette-walnut-pea-pesto-recipe/ju4lzqcd.

Working Out While Intermittent Fasting | Prospect Medical Systems. (n.d.). Www.prospectmedical.com. https://www.prospectmedical.com/resources/wellness-center/working-out-while-intermittent-fasting

Yeh, M. (2014). *Fettuccine Carbonara With Green Beans* — molly yeh. molly yeh. https://

mynameisyeh.com/mynameisyeh/2014/8/fettuccine-carbonara-with-green-beans.

Zinczenko, D., & Goulding, M. (2018). *Quick Chicken Burger With Sun-Dried Tomato Aioli Recipe* | Eat This Not That. https://www.eatthis.com/chicken-burger-sun-dried-tomato-aioli-recipe/.

Printed in Great Britain
by Amazon

69646127R00104